Get Real

Small Steps, Real Food, Big Change

MARY PRATT, NTP, BCHN & AMY YATES, BS, NTP

Dedication

For Rich, Alec, Derrick and Casey - I love you, Mary.

For Jerod, Allie, Landon and Kate with much love, Amy.

Here's what clients who've embarked on the Get Real transition with Amy and Mary through private nutrition counseling are saying...

"Working with Amy was a life changing experience! The education I received on not trying to diet but making healthy lifestyle choices has changed the way I eat, exercise, and think about things. It is not about losing weight, it's about being healthy, and naturally the weight will fall off!"

"I called Mary to work on my own nutritional needs, but what I didn't expect was a complete transformation in the way my family eats, in the way I plan and prepare food for them, and even in the money I spend on food (it's way less!). My five year old son, who has always been very picky, now asks me to prepare 'brown rice, chicken and green beans' for dinner where before he used to beg for boxed mac n cheese!"

"I didn't realize how tired I felt until I had so much more energy from changing my eating patterns. I no longer wake up feeling tired or crash during the afternoon. I'm not constantly reaching for snacks and coffee. A result that was most surprising was that I ended up losing 10 pounds over the five weeks (with Mary), without even trying or ever feeling hungry."

"When my husband and I began our journey with Amy, we knew we had to make some changes in our diet because of family histories, but we didn't know quite where to start. She provided the support and encouragement we needed to begin transforming our overall health through education, delicious, do-able recipes and supplements. We are forever grateful for the ways she has empowered us to make positive choices that impact our family on a daily basis!"

"It's a Lifestyle, not a diet. Jump in unconditionally, the program works. I started hoping to lose a few pounds, I lost 12 pounds and gained clear skin, clear mind and a clear understanding of what foods don't feel good for my body. The positives of Mary's program are body and food awareness, you will feel great (no more cravings), tips and tweaks, learned how to pay attention at the grocery store and you will discover new foods that taste great and satisfy."

"I had no idea how important making the right food choices are. Working with Amy has totally transformed me, I feel better than I ever have."

"I kept hearing how bad sugar and high-carbohydrate diets were and wanted to see if I could physically feel differently by cutting out the sugar and eating real whole foods. The result was nothing short of spectacular. I didn't realize how tired I felt until I had so much more energy from changing my eating patterns. I no longer wake up feeling tired or crash during the afternoon. I'm not constantly reaching for snacks and coffee. A result that was most surprising was that I ended up losing 10 pounds over the five weeks, without even trying or ever feeling hungry. – Thank you Mary"

"Working with Amy has been so easy. She truly understand life and is gentle to enough to suggest small changes that really work. For two years now me and my family have followed this lifestyle plan. It now is just a way of life."

"I began working with Amy Yates, who prayerfully began to realign my meal plan for optimum wellness. She gently incorporated a supplement regime. 25 years ago, I had my gallbladder removed and had never been told that I needed to take bile salts. That one addition brought immediate digestive relief. I was sick and tired of being sick and tired and did precisely as Amy instructed. In one month, I went an entire week without coughing. Global travel has made strategic eating challenging , but after working with Amy for several months, I am able to restore quickly without resorting to injections. Amy's dedication to wellness through healthy live foods and her encyclopedic knowledge of why and how certain sup-plements and foods work has opened my eyes and restored my health."

"I started this journey not only overweight but also unhealthy and I am amazed how my perception of food has changed over the last eight months. Now, it is very common to hear, 'you look younger,' 'you look good,' 'what are you doing, you look great!' These comments relate to the quality of my food intake and the increase in water consumption. Mary has gently led me to make wiser choices and therefore, has shown me how to live a healthier life. This path is a huge blessing, I am so thankful to be living a healthier lifestyle and I look forward to reaping more benefits as I continue my journey."

CONTENTS

INTRODUCTION
Why Get Real?

What do we mean when we say Get Real? First, we're talking about choosing food that's grown traditionally, prepared simply and that's nourishing for the body. But we're also talking about small, simple steps that are manageable for you and your family's busy lifestyle. Getting Real is about eating healthier, but it's also about taking stock of your family's wellbeing, finding balance and supporting a gradual lifestyle transition together.

We're working mothers who have active kids and busy lives that don't allow us to wear aprons and prepare gourmet meals. We understand your demanding lifestyle, because we are living it, too. We're also real food advocates who know firsthand that we can't just ignore nutrition and not expect consequences. This book is our solution to that conundrum; it's a lifestyle transition we've guided countless clients through and have also accomplished with our own families. The Get Real plan is a way to reap the dramatic benefits from a real foods diet amid a hectic, demanding, modern family life.

We also know how overwhelming the idea of healthful eating can seem, how nutrition can get pushed to the bottom of the pile, diets easily taken up, and then later forgotten. But it doesn't have to be like that! In fact, a real foods lifestyle like the Get Real plan can be a simple and liberating way to come together as a family and practice mindfulness, declutter your pantry and your lives and get healthy together.

Yes, the Get Real plan is healthier—but it's also simpler. The pages ahead provide realistic, affordable ways for families to make these changes without ever feeling overwhelmed. Remember, it's a lifestyle transition. The Get Real plan is a slow process that introduces big changes simply with a series of small steps.

The Plan: TAKE SMALL STEPS TOWARD REAL CHANGE.

OUR GET REAL PLAN INCLUDES:

- A guide to make a successful transition to a real-food, nutrient-filled lifestyle
- An explanation of why these real foods are beneficial
- A day-by-day and week-by-week guide to help create new habits
- Easy-to-understand facts to support each recommendation, because education is the key to success
- A summary of the effects of refined and processed foods in our bodies
- Meal plans and easy-to-follow recipes
- Special bonus topics
- Motivation for improved health

These signs will help you navigate through Get Real, here is a short explanation of their meaning.

We are firm believers in Small Steps to Big Change. Throughout the book we include quick simple instructions to follow and over time will lead to transformation.

We are excited to guide you and share our experiences. These are examples of our own process as well as challenges for you to reflect on.

THE GET REAL STORY

We're both holistic nutritional therapists with active client bases and busy families. A few years ago, we found ourselves in Austin, TX at our first Nutritional Therapy Conference. We immediately connected around a shared passion for holistic nutrition, and similar roles as busy moms with a sincere desire to do better by ourselves and our families.

Little did we know that our studies would open our eyes to the reality of the food epidemic that our culture has fallen into, one full of processing, chemical additives, poor fats and refined sugars. As we learned more and more about how to support proper nutrition and the vital role that real foods play in the body's wellness, we felt the need to bring this knowledge to others in a kind, compassionate way.

Today, we're doing just that with our clients, and have also successfully transitioned our own families to a Get Real lifestyle. It hasn't always been easy juggling it all, but the successes we've achieved for our clients, ourselves and our families have opened our eyes to the positive impact that a Get Real lifestyle can have on facets of our lives and health we never realized possible. From feeling more energized, to saving time and money, to even connecting more deeply with our children, these simple changes have had a truly meaningful ripple effect.

WHY REAL FOODS?

As holistic nutritional therapists, we believe wholeheartedly that education is absolutely the key to success. If you don't understand the reason you shouldn't eat that candy bar or snack on those chips, then chances are you'll probably reach for them. But when you have the information you need to understand that an apple will feed your body with the necessary fiber, vitamin C, potassium and antioxidants it needs to thrive, you're likely to snack on one instead.

Plus, if there's one thing we know as moms, it's to be prepared for that ever-present question: "Why?" Whenever a change is introduced, our children are going to demand answers and ask us until we give them a good answer (sometimes repeatedly), "But why?" So, here's why, in language for you to understand (and also in language for your kids when the time comes).

Real foods feed our bodies with the essential nutrients they need to thrive, which leads us toward optimal wellness. All of the nutrients our bodies get from real foods are essential. They work in unison throughout our system to provide regulation, lower toxicity, increase energy, gain mental clarity, lose cravings and reduce inflammation.

When we choose to eat processed and refined foods like packaged bread, cereals, chips or cookies, our bodies don't get the essential nutrients needed for optimal wellness. Those moments when we eat processed foods are missed opportunities to feed our bodies with the right nutrients, and it also loads our system with outliers like sugar, synthetic dyes and preservatives. Processed foods are not only depleted of essential nutrients, but they also inhibit the body's ability to absorb the quality foods that we do eat.

SYMPTOMS OF AN IMBALANCED DIET THAT CONTAINS TOO MANY PROCESSED FOODS:

- unsatisfied at meal time
- cravings
- lots of snacking
- low energy
- sluggishness
- brain fog
- inflammation
- digestive disturbance
- exhaustion

When you cut out processed and refined foods from your diet, and focus on nutrient-dense whole foods, the benefits to your body can be incredible.

SOME OF THE BENEFITS FROM A REAL FOODS DIET INCLUDE:

- more satisfaction
- less cravings
- fewer snacks
- restored energy
- digestive wellness
- clarity
- improved wellbeing

Plus, real foods taste better! Once we cleared the processed foods from our own diets, we couldn't believe how good real food actually tasted. After a little time, even our children began to notice the change.

 I can remember my oldest daughter jokingly telling me, "Congratulations, Mom. You've ruined instant brown sugar oatmeal for me for good." She could taste the added chemicals in those little packets after eating the real stuff for some time. - Amy

WHAT'S REAL FOOD?

There's one more question we want to answer before we get into the steps of the Get Real plan. You might be asking yourself a question something like this: "What do you mean, I'm not eating real food?" We promise, we're not getting philosophical here! Rather, when we talk about real food, we're referring to foods full of both macronutrients and micronutrients found in their most complete and unprocessed forms. Simply put, real foods are food that you can look at and tell what they once were. For example, scrambled eggs once came from an egg and applesauce once came from apples. (Even in simple foods like applesauce we may be getting several food additives or processing, so it is very important to check the label.)

CHICKEN STOCK

HOMEMADE	VS.	STORE BOUGHT
Chicken Water Salt Celery Carrots		Chicken broth, chicken fat, chicken flavor, cane sugar, yeast extract, onion powder, rosemary extract, celery, monosodium glutamate, vegetable oil, beta carotene, dehydrated mechanically separated chicken, potato starch

MACRONUTRIENTS are what our bodies need in the largest quantity. These include proteins, carbohydrates, fats and water. Some examples of foods that contain macronutrients are grilled chicken, quality cheese and vegetables.

MICRONUTRIENTS are absolutely essential to our health and wellbeing and they're also needed for proper metabolism, in a smaller quantity than macronutrients. These include vitamins and minerals. The simple example below outlines ingredients that hide in "healthy choices."

WHAT EXACTLY IS A BALANCED MEAL, ANYWAY?

When we start to look at balancing our meals to include more macronutrients we also start to include more micronutrients in our diet. Carbohydrates, proteins and healthy fats contain all the vitamins and minerals we need. When we lower the intake of processed foods and include each of these nutrients in every meal, we enable a slow-burning energy and fewer cravings. In order to feel this energy shift, we need to choose better quality carbohydrates, proteins and healthy fats.

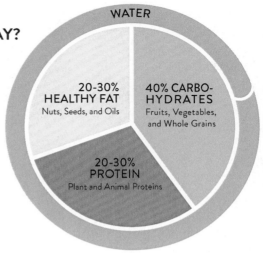

MEAL PLANS

At the end of this book, we've included four weeks of Get Real menu plans and recipes, carefully planned for a busy family life. Staying true to the "small steps, big change" philosophy, these menu plans begin with minor but impactful transitions. We've also included cleaner menus for when you're ready. All of these meals are made with simple, uncomplicated ingredients that you can find at your local grocery store.

HOW TO USE THIS BOOK

It's our hope that this book can be a practical resource that you use as a guide toward making real, nutritious, delicious and simple food a part of your family's day-to-day. It's not a diet book, a 30-day solution, nor is it even a cook book. Think of it as a guide to a lifestyle transition that you can choose to use in whatever way suits your needs. We broke this book down into small doses, and encourage you to take it slow, paying attention to each chapter individually.

Please go ahead and skip to the ending! Flip through the pages to see everything we have to offer. But once you start, please don't skip weeks. Take it slow. If your family has mastered a week, then take some time to fine-tune a previous week. Together, we're creating improved day-to-day habits, which need time to become effective.

IN OTHER WORDS, SMALL STEPS = *Big Change*

Week 1: MINDFULNESS

You might have heard the word mindfulness being used in a yoga class, in the office or from a friend who practices meditation. It's a buzzword we're all hearing more and more these days. But what exactly does mindfulness mean?

In the Get Real Plan, mindfulness means simply being aware—or taking it in—without judgment. It's a gentle way to notice your habits and choices, and then to reflect upon them. Mindfulness is the very first step in the Get Real lifestyle transition, but it's also a key component of the entire Get Real plan.

While change almost always takes a tremendous effort, the Get Real lifestyle transition should be as stress-free as possible. Mindfulness is going to help with that by emphasizing small steps, reflection, non-judgment and gentleness. Week one is all about practicing mindfulness, but there will continue to be room for mindfulness throughout the Get Real Plan. This will allow us to take the transition slowly, gently and keep it stress-free.

START WITH MINDFULNESS

For the first week of the Get Real plan, you won't need much. Just a heightened sense of your surroundings, an attitude of non-judgment and a few minutes at the end of the day for your Get Real Reflection.

Each day, you will choose one area of your lifestyle where you will practice mindfulness. You'll spend time noticing and becoming more aware of the choices being made in your home by you and your family members. Simply starting to pause and take notice will bring awareness to the areas that may need more attention, and shed light on the reasons behind your choices.

What Does Mindfulness Have to Do With Food?

So often, our choices and actions stem from subconscious habits. The definition of subconscious is being unaware. Why are we unaware? Distractions, stress, general busyness. All of these factors have a negative impact, taking our thoughts away from the moment. The Get Real goal is to sit while eating, eat slowly, read labels, taste food, notice how certain foods make us feel and to notice how diet creates energy shifts. These are not attainable when we are following distractions. When we start to practice mindfulness we pay attention, and our choices have more purpose. We become aware.

PRACTICE NON-JUDGMENT

One of the key factors in mindfulness is the absence of judgment. This is very important! We don't ever want you to be hard on yourself, judge your choices or write a list of areas "for improvement."

One thing we've noticed through the years of working with busy clients who juggle family life and careers is that we're all so hard on ourselves! Many of our clients come to us feeling down about their choices, acting as their own harshest critics. Parents especially set impossible standards for their lifestyles as they juggle careers, pressure to look fabulous and the drive to be the world's best parent, too. We ask you to reject those pressures, and to treat yourself gently instead. In the Get Real plan, there's room for mistakes. Everything is taken slowly, and each lapse is a chance for learning, never an opportunity to criticize yourself.

Your week of mindfulness may draw up many realizations that could overwhelm you as you examine them. Don't use these realizations to judge yourself or those around you! It's about reflecting, noticing ... and acknowledging. It's not even about change at this point. That change will come gradually as you progress through the Get Real plan and practice continued mindfulness. If you feel overwhelmed, take a break and remind yourself to let go of the urge to judge.

Day 1: THOUGHTS

Just notice. That is all you need to do today. As you go through your day, start to pay attention to your thoughts. Thoughts, energy, emotions and choices often stem from patterns of subconscious habits of behavior and responses. How many choices are you making out of habit?

SOME EXAMPLES OF CHOICES YOU MAKE OUT OF HABIT COULD INCLUDE:

- Reaching for a sweet snack during an afternoon slump in energy
- Ordering pizza as a way to celebrate the end of a long week
- Checking your e-mail first thing in the morning
- Turning on the television while you eat dinner
- Taking your breakfast on the go

HERE ARE SOME QUESTIONS TO ASK YOURSELF TODAY:

- How often do you turn to social media for entertainment?
- Are you mindlessly turning to social media any time you have a spare minute?
- Are your children finding down time on a daily basis?
- Does down time always include video games or screen time?

JUST NOTICE.

*As you tune in today and start to observe your choices, please keep judgments aside. This can be challenging, but wait. **Small steps will come to great change.** Today, just be mindful.*

Day 2: MOVEMENT

Spend the day reflecting on the ways you get your heart rate up. What type of activity or movement is a part of your day? Households can be very active these days, but notice if you and your family are able to fit in exercise.

Maybe your children are exercising a ton with their sports teams, while you and your spouse are sitting on the sidelines. Notice: Is there a track near the field that you can walk or run around while they practice or warm up? Maybe you get an exercise video in while your little children watch a cartoon. Notice: Is there an exercise video you can do together? Maybe you're tracking your steps with a fitness device, but never getting out of breath when you walk. Can you incorporate some hills, or pick up the pace? Today we are reflecting on all the different types of movement we engage in, and noticing opportunities to incorporate more of it into our days.

HERE ARE SOME QUESTIONS TO ASK YOURSELF TODAY:
- Do you consider your kid's extracurricular activities as your own?
- Did you and your children get outside today?
- When you sit, are you frequently at a computer or slumped on the couch?
- Is your core being activated with good posture?
- Do you find yourself looking for 'comfortable' clothes more often?
- How much time are you spending in the car?

JUST NOTICE.

Which physical activities do my family enjoy? Which ones do I enjoy? How can I start to incorporate them into our days, or our week?

Day 3: TAKE OUT

Pay attention to where you are eating. Did most of your meals this week come from a restaurant, or did you prepare them at home? Just notice, and then tally up the number of times you ate out. This includes take out, dining out, driving through and it also includes stops at your favorite coffee shop for a pick-me-up.

HERE ARE SOME OF THE QUESTIONS TO ASK YOURSELF TODAY:
- How much money did I spend on eating out?
- How much money did I spend coffee shops this week?

- What did I like about eating out?
- What didn't I like about eating out?
- How did eating out make me feel, versus eating a home-cooked meal?

Notice the number of meals you and your family ate out this week, and anything that surrounded those decisions, whether it was due to a tight schedule, an empty pantry or simply a habit.

 Do I enjoy take out or do I find it to just be the 'easiest' option? What are some of the factors that lead my family to eat out, or order take out?

Day 4: WATER

Today, pay attention to your beverage consumption, and particularly how much water you drink. What you drink can be tied to subconscious habits perhaps more than any other aspect of your lifestyle. For example, if you have a big presentation or a busy morning, do you make sure to drink extra coffee? If it's a Friday night or you are out on the weekend, do you consume alcohol? And what about with your family? What sort of habits are already formed when it comes to the beverages shared during meals? As you begin to notice these habits and associations, also notice opportunities to choose water over other beverages. Notice how certain beverages make you feel, or affect your children's behavior. Notice how water makes you all feel and act, too. And most of all, notice when you are thirsty.

HERE ARE SOME QUESTIONS TO ASK YOURSELF TODAY:
- How many glasses of water am I drinking? How much water is my family drinking?
- Are we counting other beverages as water?
- How many cups of coffee and tea am I drinking today?
- How many energy drinks and Gatorades are being consumed by my family today?

Be mindful; there's no need to change anything yet. (Although you might want to go pour yourself a glass of water as you prepare to reflect.)

 Do I recognize when I'm thirsty? Does my family drink water throughout the day, and what is the most popular beverage in my household?

Day 5: SLEEP

What does sleep look like in your home? For parents—especially those with little kids—this can be a loaded question. So many factors may affect a family's sleep patterns, from busy schedules to a baby's sleep patterns, to even the places where we sleep. Did you know that what you eat can affect your sleep patterns, too? While we can train our bodies to function on very little sleep, the long-term effect of not resting properly causes stress in the body. Take notice of your sleep patterns this week, along with the patterns of each member of your family.

SOME QUESTIONS TO ASK YOURSELF TODAY:

- How much sleep are you and your children getting each night?

- Are you able to fall asleep, but do you wake up during the middle of the night?

- Did you sleep less than eight hours last night? Why?

- When your alarm goes off in the morning, are you able to wake up?

Reflect further by comparing the hours each family member spent to the chart[1] on the right.

RECOMENDED SLEEP

AGE GROUP		NEEDED	
Newborns	0-3 Months	14-17	Hours
Infants	4-11 Months	12-15	Hours
Toddlers	1-2 Years	11-14	Hours
Preschoolers	3-5 Years	10-13	Hours
School-Age Children	6-13 Years	9-11	Hours
Teenagers	14-17 Years	8-10	Hours
Young Adults	18-25 Years	7-9	Hours
Adults	26-64 Years	7-9	Hours
Seniors	65 and Older	7-8	Hours

Remember, this week's goal is to be mindful. Don't make any sudden changes, and certainly don't go enforcing an earlier household bedtime immediately. Simply observe the way you're all sleeping, and reflect upon it.

Day 6: SPENDING

Let's take a look at how much money you spend on food. Most people believe that transitioning to a Real Foods diet will cost a lot of money. This is your chance to reflect upon the amount you already spend on food.

Take out a bank statement and add up your grocery bill for the week or month, including all the times you eat out and all of your quick stops for coffee or snacks. Sometimes it's tough to be honest when we reflect upon the money we spend. In this case, the facts are important. So get out your calculator, and keep a tally of all the money you spent on food this month. This figure will come in handy later, too.

Just reflect. Don't go instituting a budget or changing the way you shop just yet. This is a time to consider your spending and investigate the facts.

---

1   National Sleep Foundation."National Sleep Foundation Recommends New Sleep Times." Washington. D.C.: National Sleep Foundation, 2 February 2015. Web. 13 December 2016.

ASK YOURSELF THESE QUESTIONS TODAY:

- How much is your weekly grocery bill?
- Which type of food do you spend the most on at the store (packaged goods, frozen foods, produce, meat or dairy)?
- Are there local shops that you might be able to incorporate into your shopping routine, like farmers markets or farm stands during certain seasons?
- Did you buy food items just because they are on sale, regardless of nutritional value?

 Get a good understanding of your true food and drink cost.

Day 7: FOOD JOURNAL

Starting tomorrow, each family member will begin to keep a seven-day food journal. Each family member should keep a record of everything that goes into his or her mouth for one full week. Let's keep this fun and honest, leaving judgments aside. It's time for the transition to begin.

But first, be mindful about the process! The goal is to be gentle in both speech and actions, judgment cast aside. For example, you may recognize your kids eat too many chips as you work on their food journals. Instead of taking all of the chips away, allow space for the transition. Give it time. If chips are a staple, then maybe add a fruit along with them. Your children can keep enjoying the chips, just in a smaller portion. As we progress through the Get Real plan, we will help you understand the "why" behind these changes. For now, just become aware.

 Just check in with how you feel. Were any of your observations from this week surprising?

Parents of Adolescents: *The food journal is not something we can push on young adults. While the goal is to make everyone more aware of their eating, there is a fine line between awareness and obsession. Take a minute to think about your approach to this with your kids. Especially if your children are older, a food journal might not be the best way to track what they eat. Consider casual conversations, observation or a gentle talk about choices they make. We find that it works well to remind our adolescents that these choices are theirs to make as individuals.*

FOOD JOURNALS

DAY	BREAKFAST	LUNCH	DINNER
1	Quaker Apples & Spice Instant Oatmeal, Aloe Juice **Notes:** LET'S SWAP OUT THOSE INSTANT OATS FOR SOME PROPERLY PREPARED OATS. CHECK OUT OUR RECIPE FOR HOMEMADE REAL OATMEAL ON PAGE 108.	Chocolate/Espresso Cookie, Aloe Juice **Notes:** ALOE JUICE CAN BE GREAT FOR THE GUT. GOOD CHOICE. LOOKS LIKE YOU'RE ON THE GO! TRY TO PREP A GET REAL BROWN BAGGED LUNCH AHEAD OF TIME, INSTEAD OF CHOOSING A COOKIE WHEN YOU'RE IN A RUSH.	½ cup White Rice and Chicken Curry **Notes:** CHICKEN CURRY SOUNDS GREAT! LET'S ADD A GREEN SALAD. AND DON'T FORGET TO ADD A HEALTHY SNACK INTO YOUR DAY. TRY A PIECE OF FRUIT IN BETWEEN YOUR MEALS.
2	Quaker Lower Sugar Maple & Brown Sugar Instant Oatmeal **Notes:** EVEN THOUGH YOUR INSTANT OATMEAL HAS LOWER SUGAR, IT PROBABLY HAS OTHER PRESERVATIVES IN IT. IF YOU MAKE A BIG BATCH OR REAL OATMEAL EARLY IN THE WEEK, YOU'LL HAVE LEFTOVERS TO HEAT UP QUICKLY— JUST LIKE INSTANT! ARE YOU DRINKING MUCH WATER THROUGHOUT THE DAY?	½ Chicken Salad Sandwich on Baguette, Spring Salad, Iced Green Tea **Notes:** LOOKS GOOD! CHECK OUT OUR EASY HEALTHIER VERSION OF CHICKEN SALAD ON PAGE 112. CHICKEN SALAD GOES GREAT ON A RICE CAKE IF YOU WANT TO TRY SOME BREAD ALTERNATIVES, TOO.	1/2 Chicken Salad Sandwich, Milk, 2 Turtle Brownie Cookies **Notes:** WAY TO STICK TO JUST TWO COOKIES!
3	Turtle Brownie Cookie, Milk, Aloe Juice **Notes:** NICE ALOE JUICE! LETS TRY TO INCORPORATE SOME PROTEIN INTO YOUR MORNING MEALS.	Mixed Veggies, White Rice, Side Salad with Yogurt Dressing, Orange Soda **Notes:** WAY TO GO WITH THE VEGGIES AND SALAD. LET'S SET A GOAL TO BALANCE OUR MEALS A LITTLE BETTER TO GET RID OF THOSE SUGAR CRAVINGS. ADD PROTEIN OF CHOICE.	Turtle Brownie Cookie, Milk
4	Shredded Wheat and Blueberries, Coffee **Notes:** TRY SOME ALMOND MILK WITH YOUR CEREAL NEXT TIME. WAY TO ADD IN SOME BERRIES!	Couple of Slices of Brisket, Broccoli, Fried Okra and Potatoes, Corn Bread	Salad with Greens, Tomatoes and Grilled Chicken, Black Bean and Baked Chips

Week 2: HYDRATION

Everything that nourishes can also heal. (That's what the Get Real plan is all about.) Another way we like to put this: "Food is medicine."

But among all nutrients – perhaps all substances of any kind – water is unsurpassed in its powerful healing ability. Think about all the ways we use water beyond drinking it. From hot tubs to steam saunas, to swimming laps and baptism, we turn to water for healing and rejuvenation. The mere sight of water or the sound of the ocean can relieve stress and help alleviate the after effects of trauma. Water is essential to our very being.

Last week, you practiced mindfulness around your family's water consumption. This week, we'll build on those observations while setting a goal to get everyone in your household to drink more water.

A NOTE ABOUT DRINKING WATER ON THE GO

Wait! Before you run out and buy everyone expensive canteens, keep reading. We're going to suggest something a little radical: Start with disposable water bottles. Remembering to drink water all day long is a really big step. Add to that filling, keeping track of and cleaning a fancy new canteen for each of your family members? Chances are ... someone's going to lose their water bottle, and motivation may take a hit, too.

Don't worry, it will only be for one or two weeks. Next time you're at the big box store, stock up on bulk bottled water and store it somewhere cool and easy to access. This way, everyone can grab a bottle and go about their business, staying hydrated and practicing the habit, without any trips to the lost-and-found.

After one or two weeks of the Get Real approach to drinking more water, you'll make the transition to canteens for you whole family. Your carbon footprint will even out, we promise!

Day 1: CALCULATE HOW MUCH WATER YOU NEED

Today you'll calculate each family member's water needs. Try this simple math equation to get a baseline for daily water consumption requirements.

Divide your weight (in lbs.) by half.
That number is the amount of ounces of water you need as a baseline.
Add all of your diuretics[2] up (in ounces) and double that number.
Add the doubled diuretics total to the baseline water ounce total.
That's how much water you need![3]

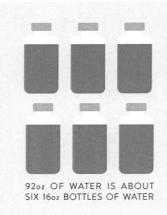

92oz OF WATER IS ABOUT
SIX 16oz BOTTLES OF WATER

EXAMPLE:

Jane weighs 120 pounds

$$\frac{120 \text{ POUNDS}}{2} = 60 \text{ OUNCES PER DAY}$$

Jane drinks 2 cups of coffee (16 ounces)

16 x 2 = 32

60 + 32 = 92

JANE NEEDS 92 OUNCES PER DAY

Now you're ready to begin sipping throughout the day! Start to track your water intake in your food journal. Lastly, take notice. Proper hydration will bring noticeable positive changes.

Keep this number in the back of your mind, and shoot for it throughout the day. Give each of your family members their numbers, too. For younger children, we recommend showing what that amount of ounces looks like (for example, show them a half-gallon carton of milk if they need 60 ounces a day).

Day 2: THE BENEFITS OF WATER

Our body composition is 65-75% water. Our body does not make water. We need to consume water daily to support our system.

You know how much water everyone needs. Next you'll need the answer to that inevitable question coming your way: "Why?"

Water does so much to optimize the way our bodies work. When you find yourself wondering what exactly it is that water does (or curious little voices asking you) refer to this handy list of its properties:

---

2   Coffee, tea, soda, energy drinks and alcohol are all diuretics.

3   It is not recommended to exceed 100 ounces/day because it can cause stress on your kidneys.

WATER

BENEFITS

Promotes Cellular Hydration

Regulates Body Temperature

Removes Waste

Flushes Toxins

Transports Nutrients

Cushions Bones and Joints

Delivers Oxygen to Your Organs

Lubricates Joints

Empowers The Body's Natural Healing Process

Some of the physical results you will feel after a week spent drinking the right amount of water include:

Increased Energy

Clear, Bright Skin

Weight Loss

Curbed Cravings

Better Mood

Less Fatigue

Fewer Headaches

More Focus

EVEN MORE REASONS TO DRINK UP...

Without water, we basically dry ourselves out. The technical term for that is dehydration and its effects can be either mild or extreme. Short-term signs of dehydration include:

Headache • Digestive Support • Hormone Balance • Constipation •

Achiness • Brain Fog • Tiredness

LONG-TERM DEHYDRATION CAN RESULT IN CHRONIC HEALTH ISSUES LIKE:

Adult Onset Diabetes

Arthritis

Asthma

Back Pain

Cataracts

Chronic Fatigue

Colitis

Constipation

Headaches

Heartburn

High Blood Pressure

Notice if you feel any of the above signs of dehydration. (If you do, drink a glass of water.)

Day 3: LET'S TALK ABOUT SODA

We've established how beneficial and essential water is for our bodies and wellness. But what about all the other stuff you drink in a day, especially soda?

Let's review Day 4 from our week of Mindfulness (see page 20). Did you gain an understanding about your family's beverage consumption? What other drinks did you notice playing a big role in your family's diet? If your family tends to drink soda, it's time to begin to wean off of it.

Remember, this is a lifestyle transition. The goal is to eventually drink no soda, but this is only week two. We're not going to burn any bridges just yet!

During your transition period, you will want to get rid of all the soda you have in your house. When you're at the grocery or big box store, stock up on those disposable water bottles and skip the carbonated stuff. (Notice that your bill will be lower as a result.)

For now, sodas can be allowed at restaurants. But no refills! Be advised, if you have teens they will have more freedom to get soda on their own. A discussion about soda and some of the negative effects (see below) can help keep your teenagers aware of their choices, and maybe even guide them to Get Real when they're out with their friends.

WHY NO MORE SODA?

They're probably going to ask you ... so here's your short answer: Soda is loaded with sugar. A 12-ounce coke has 39 grams of sugar in it. This is equivalent to eating 9 sugar cubes. And most of the time a soda at a restaurant is double that size or more.

Soda offers absolutely no beneficial nutrients. Consuming soda not only adds toxins like sugar, caffeine and chemicals to our bodies, but it also makes our systems work harder to eliminate those (and other) toxins. When we drink soda daily, our system gets bogged down with stress and toxins and causes dehydration unless replenished with water.

Does this mean diet soda is OK? No, instead of adding sugar, diet sodas add even more chemicals, which continue to be a burden on the system.

 Do not buy soda at the grocery store this week.

To rid our family of our soda drinking habits, we decided to incorporate a "two sodas per week" rule. Like most families, we kept finding these sugary drinks everywhere (church events, sporting events, school functions, grandparents' house, and of course endless refills at restaurants). So our solution was to let the kids know they could have sodas, but only two per week. They could also choose one refill at a restaurant, or one canned soda. No big swigs (believe me they tried). Now, at first this will take some guidance and gentle reminders to help your kids be mindful, but eventually it will stick. - Amy

My boys are constantly offered soda at different events. Because they are teenagers, it's less about me telling them than suggesting limitations on this. I highly encourage them to have no refills at restaurants and only one (or no) soda each week. - Mary

Parents of Adolescents: *You may gently help your teen-aged children understand why soda is not good for them and leave it at that for now. Let this be about helping them to get water in, rather than focusing too much on the negative. Remember that the goal is small steps to big change. Notice when your child has water and encourage that, rather than speaking negatively when they choose something else.*

Day 4: COFFEE AND GROWN-UP DRINKS

No worries. We promise we won't ask you to stop drinking it! But this is a good time to ask yourself a few questions about your relationship with coffee. We're all about transitions here, and we would never ask you to go cold turkey on caffeine, especially if you have busy children and a busy schedule.

Still, if you saw the name of Day 4 and immediately wanted to skip it, then that might be the first sign that your relationship with coffee needs to shift. Let's pay attention to how you're using coffee throughout the day. Some questions to ask yourself include:

- Can I get up without having a cup?
- Do I find myself using coffee as a middle-of-the-day stimulant?
- Does coffee serve as a digestive stimulant for me?
- Am I adding a sweetener or choosing lattes over regular coffee?

The pros and cons of coffee have been explored in detail in countless studies, many times with contradictory findings. Here's what the Get Real plan believes:

- Coffee is for adults. Young children and adolescents don't need the added stress that coffee puts on their ever-changing and growing bodies.
- Coffee often has a very high amount of pesticides. We recommend using organic coffee at home.
- It's a healthy goal to drink two cups, or 16 ounces, or less each day. And on a regular basis, we recommend avoiding coffee after noon.

HOW COFFEE MAY BE IMPACTING YOUR BODY

Let's revisit the mindfulness we practiced around sleep last week. What was your answer to the question, "Can you get up easily?" Your answer to that question may be tied to your need to get out of bed and go directly to the coffee pot. That's because our hormones are impacted by the amount of coffee we drink. If we have too much caffeine, it can raise our cortisol levels, which plays a huge role in our energy and sleep patterns. When our hormones are not regulated we will also start to feel more cravings for stimulants and food.

A note about digestion and coffee: The digestive system should not need the help of coffee to help regulate as long as the body is properly hydrated. Starting the day with water is the best way to keep things flowing, and then enjoy your coffee.

There's a big difference in straight black coffee and a 30 ounce caramel macchiato. Let's compare the ingredients in the labels to the right.

COFFEE

HOMEMADE

VS.

Black Coffee

Coffee
Water

STORE BOUGHT

Caramel Macchiato

Milk, brewed espresso, vanilla syrup, sugar, water, natural flavors, potassium sorbate, citric acid, corn syrup, high fructose corn syrup, sugar, butter, heavy cream, nonfat dry milk, salt, distilled monoglycerides, soy lecithin, caramel color

 If you're not ready to give up that beloved coffee drink, we understand. Try downsizing instead. Use a whole milk over two percent, stay away from soy, ask for one less pump of syrup or order a smaller size. These are all simple ways to Get Real slowly but surely.

MORE SMALL STEPS YOU CAN TAKE STARTING TODAY

You can bring your caffeine levels down to more manageable levels that are less stressful on your system with small steps like:

- Replacing an afternoon cup of coffee with a green tea
- Replacing caffeinated teas when possible with herbal varieties (chai rooibos & lemon ginger)
- Downsizing as a rule from a venti to a tall when you get your coffees on the go
- Choosing straight coffee or iced coffee over flavored coffee drinks that come laden with sugar and cream

Day 5: SPORTS DRINKS AND INFUSED OPTIONS

The options for boosting the flavor of water are everywhere. From individually packaged sugar-free powders to concentrated teas and even Gatorades, supermarkets are full of ways to make hydration a lot less healthy. Marketing has caught on that the general public recognizes we are consuming too many sodas and sweet fruit juices. But these water-enhancing flavorings are still not the best choice for our bodies. While many options are now sugar free, often those options contain some form of alternative sweeteners that can be even worse for us than an actually sugary drink. So let's skip all the water additives, stick to plain water and add a bit of fresh lemon or fruit to boost the flavor.

 If your kids are asking for something sweet, try diluting a little fresh or 100% juice with water and allow them to enjoy this as a treat (but not as a habit). If you're needing something else for yourself, try the juice or enjoy an herbal iced tea.

What Are Electrolytes? *Electrolytes are minerals in the body that have an electric charge like sodium, calcium, potassium, chlorine, phosphate and magnesium. Maintaining the right balance of electrolytes helps the body's blood chemistry, muscle action and other processes. Electrolytes also aid in the retention and replenishment of fluids. This is necessary during and after exercise due to all the fluid loss from the hard work and sweat. These minerals also play a large role in our muscle contraction and relaxation. Replenishing is essential, but not in the form that is offered by replacement drinks. Replacement drinks contain high amounts of sugar or chemicals, which actually dehydrate our system.*

Get Real Sports Drink Replacement
*Combine filtered water with a dash of sea salt and sliced oranges or lemon.
(Add a teaspoon of raw honey for some added energy for longer events.)*

Day 6: WATER QUALITY

Unfortunately, making sure we're getting enough water isn't the only hurdle. It's absolutely important that we get good quality water as well. Water is primarily used to flush our systems, but what happens when the water we're using adds more toxins?

Unfortunately, contamination of tap water is a reality. This can cause issues especially for young children, elderly, and those who deal with a compromised immune system.

Our recommendation is to find a quality filter for our homes, seeking clean and safe alternatives whenever possible.

In fact, we challenge you to go a few weeks without drinking unfiltered tap water and then try it.

You will be able to taste the additives and chemicals in it.

What water is the best water for my family?

This is a very tough question: Several water bottle companies are simply tap water from other cities, so we can't rely on bottled water to be the best alternative. Our suggestion is to do a little research about the water quality in your community and the alternative sources available to you. We understand that you probably aren't reading your local water report (it's actually required by law to be sent to every home in the U.S.).

THINGS TO LOOK FOR IN YOUR LOCAL WATER REPORT INCLUDE

- Metals such as lead, mercury and cadmium
- Overabundance of iron or aluminum
- Fecal matter
- Prescription medications
- Pesticides

Certain areas have natural spring water sources or use reverse osmosis to guarantee quality. The only downfall to reverse osmosis is that while it does remove chlorine, fluoride, bacteria, parasites, and heavy metals, it does not guarantee the removal of solvents in the water.[4]

For more information and resources visit www.watercure.com and to find the best quality filter visit EWG.org.

Day 7: AM I HUNGRY OR THIRSTY?

Did you know that our brain tissue is made up of 85 percent water? This is important information when thinking about energy, hydration and hunger. If the body is lacking hydration and nutrients, neurotransmitters send messages out to try to receive what it needs. When this signal is sent regarding water, many times we misread it, thinking our body is hungry. The reality is, we might just be thirsty.

This misinterpretation of our brain's messages can easily lead to more food consumption, weight gain and dehydration.

How do I know if I'm hungry or thirsty?

Next time you feel 'hunger' between meals – STOP. Go to your filtered water source, pour a glass of water and drink it. Wait 10 minutes and check back in with your body. You may have already forgotten about the urge to eat, or maybe you're ready to have a much lighter snack with an additional glass of water.

When we continue to consume soda, coffee drinks or excessive food we can quite easily become dehydrated. That's when signals start to become chaotic. When we answer the body's requests

---

4   Your Bodies Many Cries for Water- F.Batmangheldi, M.D.

with a glass of water, we can help calm the signals down and feed the body what it needs. Remember, water is essential to our system and we need to replenish from an outside source.

 Start your day with a glass of water before anything else (even before you drink coffee).

 As you spend this week overhauling the ways you and your family consume water, look back on the changes you've experienced. Jot down anything that strikes you as significant, whether it's less snacking, more room in the fridge or a clearer complexion. Take it in, discuss it with your family and remember that water is essential.

Week 3: BREAKFAST

Why is breakfast so important to the Get Real plan? To put it simply, breakfast optimizes metabolism. Metabolism is the way our bodies turn food into energy. When we sleep, metabolism slows way down because the body needs to do less.

When we eat first thing in the morning (or "break the fast"), we initiate the breakdown of food into energy again, and what we eat has a direct effect on how well the body can do that. Starting the day off with some healthy choices helps stabilize our appetite and insulin levels.

There are plenty more reasons that breakfast is the "most important meal." It prepares us to start the day energized, sets the tone for the rest of the meal choices we make during the day, and has a real impact on our performance. There have been studies that show data concluding that children who ate breakfast had a healthier body weight and better academic performance. One study also stated that even with different qualities of breakfast, those that ate still had better nutrition than skipping.[5]

"Eating breakfast provides energy for the brain and improves learning. The gradual decline of insulin and glucose level could determine a stress response, which interferes with different aspects of cognitive function, such as attention and working memory."[6]

Despite all the reasons that breakfast matters, it's one meal that continues to overwhelm most families. That's because morning routines are often hurried and we rely on quick and convenient meal choices. We promise, a Get Real breakfast isn't complicated, it's not going to throw your morning routine off and you don't have to give up convenience. A few simple tweaks go a long way when it comes to establishing Get Real breakfast habits.

As always, remember that this is a transition! We're not going to do anything drastic. Take it slow, and feel free to hang on to some of your old favorites while you Get Real.

Day 1: BRINGING HEALTHY TO THE TABLE

Our first transition step is to begin making familiar meals, but in healthier ways. And the very first thing you need to understand is what "healthy" actually means. Our culture is full of opinions and rules on what healthy really is, and that can be so confusing. So our goal is to make this

---

5   Journal of the American Dietetic Association, Vol 105, Issue 5, May 2005, pg 743-760.

6   Gajre, N. S., et al. "Breakfast eating habit and its influence on attention-concentration, immediate memory and school achievement." Indian Pediatrics 45.10 (2008): 824.

very simple. Healthy foods are real foods and real foods are presented in their natural state.

Still confused? Ask yourself this question next time you wonder if a food is healthy. "Can I tell what it once was without reading the label?"

Thinking about this in terms of breakfast, let's take a look at a scrambled egg. Compare it to the egg beaters that come in a little carton at the grocery store and claim to be "low fat."

This example is just another reminder to Get Real. Let's work this week and commit to starting the day with more wholesome choices.

SCRAMBLED EGGS

HOMEMADE	VS.	STORE BOUGHT
Scrambled Eggs		**Egg Beaters**
Eggs		egg whites, less than 1% natural flavor, color, (includes beta carotene), spices, salt, onion powder, vegetable gums, (xanthan gum, guar gum), maltodextrin, vitamins and minerals: calcium sulfate, iron (ferric phosphate), vitamin E (alpha tocopherol acetate), zinc sulfate, calcium sulfate, calcium pantothenate, vitamin B12, vitamin B2 (riboflavin, vitamin B1 (thiamine mononitrate, vitamin B6 (pyridoxine hydrochloride), folic acid, biotin, vitamin D3, Contains: Eggs

 Boil some eggs this evening and your breakfast will be ready for the morning.

Day 2: CEREAL

"But cereal is healthy … right?"

Not exactly. While many cereals are fortified with vitamins and minerals, that is done synthetically. In the United States, it's actually required that cereal manufacturers add synthetic nutrients back into grains. That's because they initially stripped those grains of all nutrients to give them a longer shelf life. It's all part of a "process," hence the word processed! This isn't even taking into account the oils and sugars that are often added to cereal.

Yet a bowl of cereal is almost a rite of passage for a young American kid. The boxes are marketed to them, and even the organic and "all natural" options seem to draw children in, making breakfast fun. Yes, cereal is processed. It should be replaced with real foods for your entire family. That isn't going to be easy, and it might not even be 100% feasible. It's about being aware and making the transition where and when you can. Take it slow, talk to your family about Get Real breakfast options and remember this is a transition!

When I first started transitioning my family away from cereal, I still allowed the kids to have a bowl of cereal every morning, with one new rule. They had to drink a smoothie first! This way, they got some Real nutrients into their tummies first thing, and then they still got to have a bowl of cereal, which they were used to having. - Amy

See Grumpy Smoothie Tips on page 109 for ideas on breakfast smoothies for kids.

Not only did my kids eat and love cereal, but I did too. Initially, I just transitioned myself off. Cereal was a true staple in my house so we couldn't go cold turkey. I decided it would be easier to switch it to an afternoon snack a couple days a week for the boys, rather than totally eliminate it. During that time, I transitioned the boys' breakfast and eventually just stopped serving it as an afternoon snack as well. Cereal just faded away. - Mary

 Instead of cereal, choose a breakfast option that combines a protein and a healthy fat like yogurt and granola (with some fruit and cinnamon).

Day 3: GRAINS

Many popular diets eliminate grains altogether. One reason that people feel better when they get rid of grains is that they're eliminating processed foods (like cereal) and eating more real foods. The thing about grains is, our bodies need several of the essential vitamins and minerals that grains provide, particularly the B vitamins, vitamin E, iron and sustainable fiber.

We will make several recommendations on ways to locate and prepare proper grains. This is a transition. You don't need to throw everything away, just simply stop replacing old grains as they run out. As you follow the transition plan, you will see these processed choices slowly fade away.

GET REAL BREAD BUYING GUIDE

1. Look for 100% Whole Wheat or 100% Whole Grain. This contains all three parts of the wheat kernel, each containing beneficial nutrients.

2. Read the label and ask: Is there high fructose corn syrup? If yes, then skip it.

3. Read the label and ask: Are there additives? Chemicals? If yes, skip.

4. Look for minimal ingredients: Bread only needs flour, water and salt to be prepared.

Go to your pantry and read the labels on your breads and cereals. Identify any items that you won't replace.

See page 68 for more on how to read a Label.

Day 4: AND THE COW SAYS, MOO...

Dairy is a transitional food as well as a controversial food. It is also a breakfast staple. Whether it's the milk in our cereal, cream in our coffee or yogurt in our parfait, many of us rely on dairy products to start our day.

The struggle with dairy is, like many of our modern day conveniences, mass production has compromised quality. Most of the milk found in the grocery store isn't fresh and unprocessed from a reliable source.

> **Approach to dairy:** *Buy milk, yogurt and cheese in the cleanest, most uncompromised way possible and consume it in moderation.*

If you take a minute to think about it, you realize humans are the only mammals that consume dairy after being weaned.

We're not going to completely cut out dairy. But we are going to set a goal to transition to quality dairy.

UNDERSTANDING DAIRY

1. **Know what dairy is.** We instantly think of dairy and think milk, but remember there are several other foods that fall into this category, too. Dairy products include cheese, yogurts and butter. This does not include products like Velveeta or Easy Cheese, of course. These are not quite foods, but perhaps "food-like products." Laden with chemicals to get the color, texture and taste "just right," many products claim to be dairy when in fact they are barely even food. So even though we want the Get Real plan to be a slow transition, when it comes to substances like Velveeta, it is time to transition them straight into the trash.

2. **Know what quality dairy is.** The Get Real definition of quality dairy is dairy in its least processed form. Start by looking for a high-quality, organic, whole milk. Skim milk—even when it's organic— has been fortified with nutrients that were stripped in the process of eliminating its fat. If you're not comfortable drinking whole fat milk, you can dilute it at home with pure, clean water. This not only ensures the quality, but it also saves money.

3. **Understand the nutrients we get from dairy.** Dairy provides some excellent nutrition, including calcium, live probiotics, and the valuable vitamin K2 (known for calcium uptake). It's important to understand that while dairy is a great source for these nutrients, it is not the only source. A few examples of calcium sources are dark leafy greens like kale as well as broccoli and black eye peas.

Cheese should be white, not yellow. Yellow cheese lets us know something has been added. Take this easy transition step and simply start Getting Real by switching to white cheese.

A NOTE ABOUT DAIRY ALTERNATIVES

There are several dairy alternatives available and unfortunately they are not all created equal. We recommend if you choose to use nut or coconut milks that you find a full fat nut milk with no added texturizers or sweeteners.

Soy milk is not recommended in any circumstance. Soy carries compounds that interfere with the body's ability to properly digest proteins. Additionally, soy has been shown to disrupt normal endocrine function and alter estrogen activities. Finally, the majority of soy products are not real food. Soy is very refined and highly processed.

Day 5: YOUR MOST IMPORTANT RULE IS EAT REAL FOOD!

What is a Real Breakfast? As we get started with this transition, find your favorite recipe and just go for it. Where you notice processed or unreal ingredients, sub for nutrient-dense real foods like unrefined grains, fruits, vegetables, quality dairy and proteins.

This is where we need to recognize we are all individuals and have different needs. While we do recommend transitioning the processed foods out, we also recommend adding in those nutrient-dense choices. Find your favorite breakfast recipe, and start supplementing with extra nutrient-dense foods. Some examples include:

Favorite Breakfast
- Toast with butter
- Instant oatmeal
- Eggos
- Fruit-flavored yogurt
- Cereal with low-fat milk

Get Real Boost
- Ezekiel toast, almond butter
- Steel cut oats with real or frozen blueberries
- Get Real pancakes see "Oatmeal Pancakes" on page 107 for recipe
- Bulgarian yogurt with fresh fruit
- Granola, fruit and whole milk

The benefit of starting the day loaded with nutrients leaves us more satisfied and sets us up for more balanced choices throughout the day. In fact, there is something called the 'Second Meal Effect,' which aids in glucose tolerance at the following meal. Clinical nutrition states, "slow and prolonged absorption of carbohydrates at breakfast results in a slower rise in blood sugar levels, a reduced insulin response and a lessened glycemic response after lunch."[7] Translation: Choose wholesome foods in the morning and this will support you and your body's response even after your next meal.

---

7   Jeffrey S. Bland, et al, Clinical Nutrition(IFM, 2004), 35.

This is a perfect place to practice mindfulness. Notice how you feel after breakfast. Are you still hungry? Are you hungry in an hour? Satisfied until lunch? Start to take notice of these feelings and how they change as you make your Get Real substitutions.

Work with this for a couple weeks, have a few different types of breakfast and see which type gives you the best kick-start to your day!

Day 6: "BUT I'M TOO BUSY..."

We know, we get it and yes, mornings go by quickly. Let's look at some options that are superior in choice and nutrients, but just as timely as pouring a bowl of cereal. Yes, some will require prior prep time. Thinking ahead can make your mornings even simpler.

GET REAL QUICK BREAKFAST OPTIONS

- Mason Jar Oats or Crock Pot Oats, see "Overnight Oatmeal" on page 108 for recipe
- Smoothie (cut up the fruit the night before, and store it in your blender in the fridge.)
- Fruit and nuts
- Applesauce and granola
- Yogurt and berries
- Pop tart toast, see ""What Happened to Our Pop Tart? Toast" on page 110 for recipe
- Hard boiled eggs with fruit
- Egg sandwich on sourdough bread
- Leftovers (Seriously! Love cold pizza for breakfast? Try quinoa with blueberries and cinnamon. Or try savory real breakfasts ready in a zap!)
- Apple with nut butter

MAKE-AHEAD RECIPES FOR BREAKFAST ON-THE-GO

PRE-MADE GRANOLA BARS

INGREDIENTS: oats, cinnamon, salt, coconut oil, nut butter, egg

2 cups	oatmeal	Blend all ingredients together.
½ cup	nut butter	
1 teaspoon	cinnamon	Bake at 350 for 15 - 18 minutes in a parchment lined pan.
dash	sea salt	Optional add-ins: protein powder, hemp hearts, chia seeds, raisins.
2 tablespoons	raw honey	
4 tablespoons	coconut oil	
1	egg	

HEALTHY TRAIL MIX IDEAS
- Walnuts, apple chips and coconut chips
- Almonds, dried apricot and dark chocolate nibs

EGG 'MUFFINS'

INGREDIENTS: eggs, chopped onion, bacon or turkey sausage, sea salt, cayenne (optional), parchment paper muffin liners

12	eggs	Place parchment paper muffin liners in 12-muffin pan. Blend eggs with chopped onion, bacon or turkey sausage, and a dash of cayenne.
¼ cup	chopped onion	
¾ cup	bacon or sausage	
½ teaspoon	sea salt	
dash	cayenne (optional)	Pour mixture into lined pan and bake at 350 for 30 minutes.

With a little work up front, the day will start with more ease and predictability. Meals do not need to be fancy – sometimes going back to basics works best.

Time & Money Breakout

'Quick' Stop at the Coffee Shop

COST: **$7 (average receipt)**

TIME SPENT: **15 minutes in line**

OR

Coffee & Breakfast at Home

COST: **$3**

TIME SPENT: **15 minutes sitting peacefully and eating**

Day 7: "I'M JUST NOT HUNGRY IN THE MORNINGS"

Did you know waking up not hungry is linked to digestion? Our digestive systems are very active while we sleep and if we're not digesting efficiently, the food is not being broken down and assimilated. That's why you're waking up not feeling hungry.

IF YOU'RE ONE OF THE "NOT HUNGRY IN THE MORNING" TYPES, ASK YOURSELF THE FOLLOWING QUESTIONS

- Am I chewing my food well?
- Do I take my time while I eat?
- Do I stop when I feel full?
- Am I 'regular'? Do I go daily? (To the restroom, that is.)

Eating a really big dinner late in the evening could also contribute to a lack of hunger in the morning.

 Stop eating two hours before bedtime.

While in general we'd never suggest eating even if you're not hungry, when it comes to breakfast, we make an exception. Not waking up hungry is a red flag that something's going on with your digestion (a Real Foods plan will help with that) or your evening dining habits. We're going to urge you to reach for something wholesome in the morning, no matter how full you feel, to kick start your metabolism, stabilize your blood sugar levels and remain energized until your next meal.

HOW TO "BREAK THE FAST" EVEN WHEN YOU'RE NOT HUNGRY

Eat a small breakfast. We know you're not hungry, but start the day with a piece of fruit anyway. Have a healthy snack (nuts, hard boiled egg, trail mix) before lunch.

Eat regular meals throughout the day. Eat three meals a day and one or two healthy snacks rather than waiting until late afternoon and evening to consume most of your calories. You will eat less food throughout the day because you won't be as hungry.

If your schedule allows, have a bigger lunch and a lighter dinner. Notice how you feel from this shift.

 Start your day with lemon water (warm or cold).

Week 4: HEALTHY FATS

A balance of healthy fats in the diet is essential for our bodies to function properly. In fact, fats are part of every cell membrane, tissue and organ in the body. Without healthy fats, or with too many of the unhealthy kind of fats, the integrity of our cells is challenged, plain and simple. This can have a detrimental effect on health over time.

Fats do much more, too! In fact, below is a list of the many roles that healthy fats play in the body.

THE MANY FUNCTIONS OF HEALTHY FATS

Source of energy: A balance of quality fats helps to maintain a steady energy level, rather than the compromised energy level that comes from sugar/processed foods.

Inflammation management. The properties of healthy fats support the body's inflammation function, when unhealthy fats are removed.

Hormone management. Not only are hormones derived from healthy fats, but the body cannot make certain hormones without healthy fats.

Absorbing vitamins: Vitamins A, D, E & K need to be consumed with healthy fat in order to be absorbed and utilized in our systems.

Necessary for healthy liver function. Quality fats help to provide adequate consistency in bile production, thus aiding in proper digestion.

Mood balancing: A lack of quality fats in the diet has been related to an inability to focus, anxiety and depression. (Please understand that diet is just a piece of the puzzle when it comes to mood, but one worth considering.)

Removing low quality fats from your diet and incorporating quality fats with every meal will start a shift toward lowering inflammation and gaining more balance in hormones, moods, skin, and energy. Eating healthy fats is an integral step in the path toward healing and wellness.

Day 1: UNDERSTANDING YOUR FATS

Before we start transitioning, let's get a better understanding of healthy fats. Fatty acids provide a concentrated source of energy while also functioning as the building blocks of every cell membrane within the body. On the most cellular level, where disease and dysfunction begin, fat is essential for cell-to-cell communication.

The following consequences have been associated with a low or poor fat-diet.

SOURCE:
Enig, Mary G. Know Your Fats.
Bethesda: Bethesda Press 2000.

ADD	Cravings	Inflammation
Allergies	Depression	Learning disabilities
Anxiety	Digestive disorders	Skin disorders
Autoimmune disease	Infertility	Tension headaches

As you become more mindful of the healthy and not-so-healthy fats in your diet this week, remember:
- *healthy fats are essential on the most cellular level*
- *poor fats cause damage on a cellular level*

Day 2: TAKING INVENTORY OF YOUR FATS

Not all fats are beneficial and some can be harmful. Head over to your pantry and check the packaged goods, oils and snacks you have there. Poor or lower quality fats are often used for preservatives to extend the shelf life of packaged goods. They can also be found in gluten free, organic and other seemingly healthy foods. The bottom line? Our bodies are not created to digest these poor fats. Breaking them down can cause long-term health ramifications.

FATS

A balance of healthy fats is essential for health and healing.

HEALTHY OPTIONS

SATURATED FATS

- Coconut oil
- Palm oil
- Grass-fed butter
- Ghee
- Chicken fat
- Raw or full fat dairy
- Eggs
- Meats/seafood

UNSATURATED FATS

- Olive oil
- Sesame oil
- Nuts and seeds
- Nut butter
- Flaxseed
- Macadamia nut oil
- Avocado
- Hemp hearts
- Wild caught fish

UNHEALTHY OPTIONS

- Margarine
- Spreads
- Canola oil
- Vegetable oil
- Soybean oil
- Grapeseed oil
- Safflower oil
- Sunflower oil
- Rice bran oil
- Shortening made from any of the oils listed above

Linolenic and alpha-linolenic acid *are two fats that are absolutely essential to incorporate into the diet. They are more commonly know as Omega-3 and Omega-6 fatty acids. The body cannot simulate these fats; they must be ingested. These essential fats can be found in cold water fish, walnuts, flax seeds and even leafy vegetables.*[8]

Hydrogenated or partially hydrogenated oils and man-made "spreads" are highly processed. Materials such as bleach and nickel are used. They oxidize easily via light, air or heat. While hydrogenated oils extend the shelf life and lower the actual fat content of a product, they're toxic for the body.

Our bodies are not created to process these manufactured fats. In addition, these poor fats have been highly correlated with obesity and a lower plasma concentration. They're also connected with cholesterol build up, weight gain and heart disease. Likewise, when we choose the proper type of fats weight loss (largely due to appetite control) and even a lower BMI result.

8   Chow CK. Fatty Acids in Foods and Their Health Implications, 2nd Edition. CRC Press, 1999; pp. 17-46.

Continue to read labels and be a wise consumer. Can you pronounce what you're reading? Do you know where these products come from?

PEANUT BUTTER CRACKERS

HOMEMADE

Organic Peanut Butter on Organic Thin Stackers

organic peanut butter: organic peanuts, sea salt

thin stackers: organic brown rice, sea salt

VS.

STORE BOUGHT

Peanut Butter Crackers

unbleached enriched flour (wheat flour, niacin, reduced iron, thiamine mononitrate {vitamin B1}, riboflavin {vitamin B2}, folic acid), peanut butter (peanuts, hydrogenated rapeseed and/or cottonseed and/or soybean oils, salt and peanut oil), soybean oil, sugar, dextrose, partially hydrogenated cottonseed oil, high fructose corn syrup, salt, leavening (baking soda and/or calcium phosphate), soy lecithin, malted barley flour

Day 3: FAT BURNER VS. SUGAR BURNER

Our metabolisms are designed to use fats for long-term energy. Often, due to our dietary choices, the body will rely on sugar rather than fat for a primary quick energy source. At Get Real, we call this type of metabolism "Sugar Burner."

Choosing sugar over quality fat actually trains the body over time to switch off its fat burning metabolism. This also aids in creating a blood sugar dysfunction cycle page 56. The Get Real goal is to reduce the higher amounts of processed, refined and sugary foods and increase some healthy fats, which will help the body transition to using fats for long-burning energy.

The body does need glucose but not in the form of processed sugar. Glucose is essential to blood sugar regulation and sustained energy levels. When sugar is over consumed, we must use stored insulin to transport glucose. Overconsumption of sugar can cause insulin reserves to tap out (more on this next week). This process is what can lead to Type 2 diabetes, where the body can't make enough insulin to transport glucose through the system properly.

GET REAL: TAKE A MINUTE TO ANSWER THE NEXT FEW QUESTIONS[10]

Do you have cravings for sweets or breads?

Does your diet consist of a large amount of processed grains and refined sugar?

Do you have insistent hunger?

Frequent snacking?

Difficulty losing weight?

Are you tired after meals?

Answering YES = Sugar Burner

Do you feel satisfied between meals?

Do you have plenty of energy?

Can you lose weight if needed?

Do you have sustained energy between meals?

Answering YES = Fat Burner

As you transition toward including more healthy fats, you will feel your energy shift to a more sustained level, you'll feel satisfied (and experience less cravings) and you'll train your body to burn fat.

Incorporate healthy fats into your snack this week. We like half of a small avocado with lemon and sea salt. Another easy go-to for kids and adults is nut butter with an apple or thin rice cake.

Day 4: SWAPPING OILS

Hopefully by now, you and your family have transitioned to eating a healthy breakfast. Does this meal contain high protein and fat content? Remember that fats give you more sustained energy, and will ensure that you're consuming the nutrients necessary to get through the day. Now that you know about that energy secret, it's time to start adding healthy fats to your Get Real breakfast. The most convenient kinds are foods that have both protein and fat like eggs, nuts and full-fat Bulgarian yogurt.

One of the easiest ways to start incorporating healthy fats into your diet throughout the day is through oil swapping. Use the chart on the next page to start getting rid of all the bad fats you unintentionally consume and get in those energy-sustaining, cell-membrane-building healthy fats!

---

9   These questions aren't diagnostic, they're simply a guideline to help you notice your food choices.

INSTEAD OF		BEST CHOICE
Cooking spray, margarine or hydrogenated oils		Coconut oil or grass-fed butter
Canola/vegetable oil		Extra virgin olive oil, ghee or coconut oil
Roasted nuts		Raw nuts
Nut butters with added oil and sugar		Simple nut butters

As you make this transition, only replenish your pantry with healthy fats. When buying oils, make sure they are packaged in a dark bottle (except for coconut oil). Once light and heat hit the oil, the chemical makeup changes. When the oils change chemically they become rancid and difficult for our body to digest.

Our goal is to help you find affordable, healthy choices. *We understand that life has its demands and finances are often one of the biggest demands. In your Get Real grocery budget, fats and oils will take a priority in spending. It's important to remember that healthy fats like avocados and oils are more expensive, but a little goes a long way.*

 Start the transition from poor quality fats to healthy fats. These healthy fats serve as nourishment, while the poor quality fats cause dysfunction.

LET'S BEGIN TO EXPERIMENT WITH HEALTHY FATS IN OUR RECIPES THIS WEEK

- Scrambling some eggs? Rather than using PAM® or margarine, indulge in some grass-fed butter or ghee.
- Dinner time? Start to integrate coconut oil or extra virgin olive oil rather than vegetable oils.
- Homemade dressing: 1 tablespoon of extra virgin olive oil (evoo), 1 tablespoon balsamic vinegar, sea salt, black pepper, a touch of raw honey (optional add ins: dijon mustard, dried herbs, garlic).

Day 5: SERVING SIZE

How much healthy fat is too much? Activity level, age, and other factors play a role in how much fat our bodies need. More important than the quantity is the quality. Once you and your family have maintained healthy fats in your diet for a while, you will begin to physically recognize the differences between good and bad fats.

As you start to incorporate the healthy fats into your diet, also recognize that everyone has different needs based on lifestyle and bio-individuality. There is no special formula. Some individuals can eat more (or less) than the amounts listed. This is where mindfulness comes into play: eat and recognize how you feel after a meal (hungry, satisfied, irritable, bloated, etc). Keeping a food journal is beneficial, especially during a transition.

SERVING SIZES   PAY ATTENTION TO LABELS AND NOTE THE SERVING SIZE

Ghee, grass-fed butter, coconut oil, EVOO	½ - 1 tablespoon
Raw nuts	¼ - 1/3 cup
Nut butters	1-2 tablespoons
Avocado	½ small or ¼ whole

Get Real Mindfulness Reminder

When eating nuts, take your serving and put the container away. This will prevent mindless eating and maintain an appropriate serving. As you're snacking on nuts, are you sitting? Are you taking your time?

MINDFULNESS CHECK IN:

Within one to three hours after a meal, place a check in the box next to any selection that applies to you. Once meals are transitioned and balanced, we will connect with more of the feelings from the blue column.

If you are experiencing more in the red column, take a look at your food journal. Look at the ways you can decrease refined carbohydrates, increase healthy fats and bring more balance (page 15) into your meals.

	GOOD FAT / CARB RATIO	**MODIFY** FAT / CARB RATIO
APPETITE, FULLNESS, SATISFACTION & SWEET CRAVINGS	☐ Feel full and satisfied ☐ No sweet cravings ☐ Not looking for more food ☐ Do not get hungry soon after eating ☐ Do not need to snack before next meal	☐ Feel physically full, but still hungry ☐ Don't feel satisfied; feel like something was missing from meal ☐ Have desire for sweets ☐ Feel hungry again soon after meals ☐ Need to snack between meals
ENERGY LEVELS	☐ Energy is restored after eating ☐ Have good, lasting sense of energy and wellbeing	☐ Too much or too little energy ☐ Become hyper, jittery, shaky, nervous or speedy
MENTAL & EMOTIONAL WELLBEING	☐ Improved wellbeing ☐ Feel refueled or restored ☐ Uplift in emotions ☐ Improved clarity of mind ☐ Normalization of thought process	☐ Mentally slow, sluggish, spacey ☐ Inability to think clearly, quickly ☐ Overly rapid thoughts ☐ Inability to focus ☐ Hypo-apathy, depression, sadness ☐ Irritability ☐ Hyperactivity ☐ Energy drop, fatigue, exhaustion, sleeplessness, drowsiness, lethargy or listlessness

CHECK ALL THAT APPLY

---

10 This chart isn't diagnostic, it is simply a guideline to help you notice and shift your food choices

Day 7: WHAT ABOUT THE KIDS?

Including quality fats and excluding poor fats is absolutely essential in every diet. During the developmental stages, there are several factors that determine the amount of fat cells each individual will have. Once we reach adulthood, our body has a set number of fat cells, which enlarge or shrink to accommodate the increase or decrease in triglyceride storage. For example, a person can lose a substantial amount of weight yet still have the same amount of fat cells. The cell itself has just shrunk in size.

It is of utmost importance that as parents we provide our children with the highest quality fats from infancy to adolescence.

During the infancy/toddler phase, parents have some control over what their children eat. Once solid food is introduced, you may begin to introduce healthy, wholesome foods and healthy fats. This is also a great time to introduce vegetables and remember – adding a healthy fat is not only delicious, but also beneficial. Don't forget baby's favorite, a mashed avocado.

Elementary years start to include of few more challenges. Packed lunches prevent access to the bad oils used in the school cafeteria. This is also a time to be a great influence in your community and lead your children by example. Advocate for reward systems other than food in the classroom and keep the party fun with activities rather than a focus on sweets. Check out our lunchbox recipe options (page 111). There are endless options of healthy, "fun" foods for kids to enjoy.

Adolescence has more challenges because of the freedom our children gain during these years. When they have lived with wholesome choices and are educated 'why' they are the best choices they are more apt to choose wisely – most of the time. It's also important for them to start experiencing on their own and they will feel the effects of healthy vs. unhealthy choices. Most adolescents will make some unhealthy choices, but their bodies will tell them when to stop. Acne may arise when their diet strays. Once an adolescent makes this connection, the healthy choice may become easier to make.

With all ages, we want you to keep offering healthy nutrients. Yes, there may be some resistance. Eventually, they will choose quality, real foods more often. We all know kids are led by example, keeping these choices on your menu will make a significant difference.

In our private practices we have both worked with teens outside of our home. As their nutritionist we took the small steps approach and shifted their diets to include healthy fats and less processed foods. Some of the effects these clients have experienced are remarkable:

- *Overall more energy*
- *No need to nap after school*
- *More endurance as an athlete*
- *Improved skin*
- *Improved concentration at school*

The shifts have brought more awareness to their choices. They feel the connection and have been motivated to keep the transitions in their lifestyle.

CHECK IN WITH BREAKFAST: How has your morning routine shifted? Are you eating more foods from home? We know it's hard to get out the door, take a look at some of our smoothie recipes (page 109) and incorporate one into your routine this week.

Week 5: SUGAR

The average American eats 130 pounds of sugar a year. This is approximately 32 tsp (160 g) of sugar every day. This is a rather large amount of sugar when you break it down like this.

Most likely, many of us are getting even more sugar than that! Sugar is hiding almost everywhere. It lurks in meals prepared in restaurants and pre-packaged foods. A flavored yogurt alone has more sugar than the recommended daily intake.[11]

When the low-fat craze started many years ago, food distributors started to remove healthy fats and increase sugar content to make products have more flavor. Our society has accepted sweetness as a norm. Instead of enjoying an occasional dessert, sweets have become a part of each meal. But a sweet tooth comes at a cost.

Sugar can be addicting, and has numerous effects on our emotional wellbeing and overall health. Get Real's goal for helping you and yours kick the sugar addiction is a gentle, yet realistic approach. We realize that as a whole most of us don't even realize the amount of sugar that we consume on a daily basis. Our first desire is for you to become aware.

Day 1: READ THE LABEL

Today, be mindful and observe how much sugar you and those in your household are consuming. Often we're simply not aware as we continue to buy the same goods each week. When you eat a prepared food, look at the label.

According to the FDA, the term "natural" can be placed on any food product that originated from nature, regardless of what has been done to it since it was in its natural state.

HERE ARE SOME THINGS TO LOOK FOR

- How much added sugar is in the product?
- Glance at the ingredients. Do you recognize the foods listed? Is sugar one of the first three ingredients?
- Take a look at the list of forms of sugar below. Are any of these hiding in your favorite products?

---

11 Yoplait™ original strawberry - 18 grams of sugar

When you're reading labels, remember that sugar can be disguised as any number of terms, including:

Agave nectar	Date sugar	Fruit juice concentrate	Muscovado
Barley malt	Demera	Galactose	Panoha
Beet sugar	Dextran	Glucose	Raw sugar
Blackstrap molasses	Diastase	Golden syrup	Rice syrup
Brown sugar	Diastatic sugar	Grape sugar	Sorghum
Cane sugar	Ethyl maltol	Honey	Sucrose
Carmel	Evaporated cane juice	Lactose	Treacle
Carob	Florida crystals	Maltodextrin	
Confectioners sugar	Fructose	Maltose	
Corn syrup			

SOURCE:
Sanfilippo, Diane. Practical Paleo. Las Vegas: Victory Belt Publishing, 2012. (99-103)

FAMILY CHALLENGE

Make this fun and light, with no judgments. At this point, it's more about mindfulness than how much sugar everyone is consuming. We are even going to recommend that you go out and purchase a container of sugar cubes for the purpose of mindfulness!

Have each family member spontaneously grab their favorite sweet treat from the kitchen. Check out the labels. Convert the grams per serving to sugar cubes (4g = 1 tsp = 1 sugar cube). This is a great visual to see how much sugar each of you are getting. As parents, we would never let our kids eat sugar cubes for breakfast before going to school, but that's what we're doing when we send them out the door with a glass of chocolate milk!

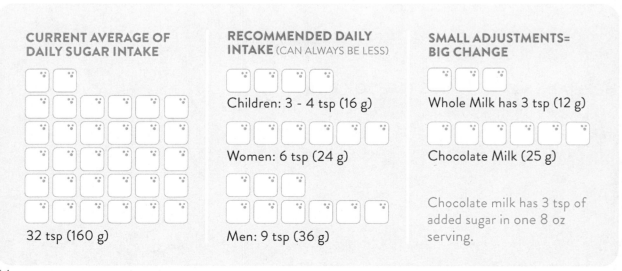

CURRENT AVERAGE OF DAILY SUGAR INTAKE

32 tsp (160 g)

RECOMMENDED DAILY INTAKE (CAN ALWAYS BE LESS)

Children: 3 - 4 tsp (16 g)

Women: 6 tsp (24 g)

Men: 9 tsp (36 g)

SMALL ADJUSTMENTS= BIG CHANGE

Whole Milk has 3 tsp (12 g)

Chocolate Milk (25 g)

Chocolate milk has 3 tsp of added sugar in one 8 oz serving.

Day 2: THE EFFECTS

Yesterday we noticed the added sugar in some of our choices. Today let's think about the effects of this added sugar.

NOTICING THE CYCLE

Eating an imbalanced diet with excess refined carbohydrates will indeed lead to stored fat, imbalance and eventually inflammation. These refined carbohydrates DO NOT satisfy. Eventually, we will feel drastic energy shifts, mood swings and cravings. At that point, our cravings will be persistent which will lead to a choice of more refined carbohydrates. A cycle is created.

Persistent sweetness from both sugar and artificial sweeteners becomes a stimulus. Our taste receptors become desensitized and we look for more sweetness.

Review the quiz "Get Real: Take a minute to answer the next few questions" on page 47 regarding our satisfaction and mood cycles. What column can you associate with the most? Making these subtle shifts in our choices can lead to big changes both emotionally and physically.

> *Remember, processed sugar has no nutritional value. That said, placing sugar restrictions in your household may cause resistance. Please remember you didn't get here overnight so please DO NOT change everything overnight.*

Side effects of removing sugar (we are speaking from experience here):

- Children and spouse may rebel.
- Withdrawals will occur (these may include headaches, crankiness and sluggishness).

THE GOOD NEWS: You have already successfully begun this transition by eliminating or reducing your family's soda consumption.

Spend the day observing any shifts in mood, energy and cravings as well as the choices that are made in your household.

SLEEP CHECK IN: In Week 1 we spent a day focusing on our sleep. Did you know our blood sugar can affect our sleep patterns? If we are choosing higher amounts of processed foods and sugar it can be too stimulating for us to get to sleep or cause some hormone fluctuation during the middle of the night and wake us up. Sleep is also a time for our bodies to regulate certain hormones, work through digestion, detoxify and support brain function.

Day 3: UNDERSTANDING THE CYCLE

While blood sugar regulation is very complicated, the goal here is to help you understand it from a nutrition aspect; this is not a diagnostic explanation.

Blood sugar dysfunction is a cycle that can be created by dietary choices, stress responses, and unfortunately, genetics. While some components of blood sugar regulation cannot be manipulated, one's diet can play a large role in balancing blood sugar. People often consume a high amount of refined carbohydrates and a low amount of healthy fats. The hormone insulin is released in order for the body to assimilate glucose (broken down carbohydrates).

The more glucose ingested, the more insulin produced.

Short-term energy becomes a constant. We are made to have longer periods of energy, but our body processes sugar/glucose quicker than proteins and fats. The body releases more insulin to manage the high amounts of ingested processed foods/sugars. Eventually, our organs stop accepting glucose, get overworked and these nutrients end up being stored as fat (fat accepts the extra 'stuff').

Our system becomes imbalanced.

Cortisol is a stress hormone that has many roles in the body such as protein breakdown, breakdown of triglycerides, and anti-inflammatory effects, the role we will focus on is Glucose Formation. If the body has excess insulin (a stressor), it creates excess cortisol. This starts to impair the delicate balance of our system, and we may experience strong cravings. This is the body's way of trying to attain balance. We may also experience drastic energy shifts.

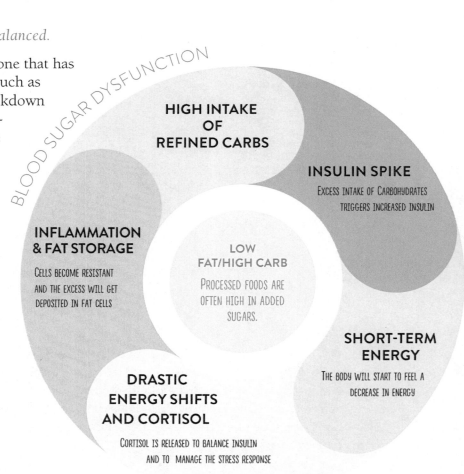

BLOOD SUGAR DYSFUNCTION

HIGH INTAKE OF REFINED CARBS

INSULIN SPIKE
Excess intake of Carbohydrates triggers increased insulin

INFLAMMATION & FAT STORAGE
Cells become resistant and the excess will get deposited in fat cells

LOW FAT/HIGH CARB
Processed foods are often high in added sugars.

SHORT-TERM ENERGY
The body will start to feel a decrease in energy

DRASTIC ENERGY SHIFTS AND CORTISOL
Cortisol is released to balance insulin and to manage the stress response

Get Real: Take a look at your food journal.
- *Does your day have large amounts of refined carbohydrates?*
- *Have you started to welcome more healthy fats?*

"Childhood obesity has more than doubled in children and quadrupled in adolescents in the past 30 years." This epidemic causes both short-term and long-term health implications. "The increasing frequency of both type 1 and type 2 diabetes in youth has been among the most concerning aspects of the diabetes epidemic." [12]

DAY 4: ADULTS

Blood sugar regulation is closely tied to hormone regulation as well as how efficiently the body absorbs nutrients. Blood sugar dysfunction is a common trigger that makes hormones volatile.

Many of the symptoms of hormone dysfunction may be familiar to you. Have you experienced bloating, hot flashes, irregular cycles, breast tenderness, headaches, fatigue, lack of libido, sleepless nights or anxiety? These aren't necessarily symptoms of aging. They could be part of the cycle of blood sugar dysfunction, and eliminated or diminished by focusing on a healthy, Get Real lifestyle. Focusing on a healthy lifestyle is the first step in regulating blood sugar and balancing hormones.

Toxins from sugar (along with processed foods and unhealthy fats) impact the liver's ability to clear out hormones. When this happens, the liver becomes overworked trying to regulate hormones. These dietary choices have a negative impact on hormones. When we continually eat sugar, our bodies are in a constant state of stress response.

GET REAL TIPS FOR HORMONE BALANCE
- Eat your veggies. Start to fill half your plate with healthy vegetables. Vegetables are filled with fiber and nutrients that balance blood sugar.
- Choose more low-sugar fruits such as berries, apples and pears. These are real foods that have lower levels of sugar, are fiber rich and help to keep insulin levels low.
- Lower your alcohol intake. The liver is designed to stop its primary functions when it becomes focused on clearing out consumed alcohol. In addition, this is broken down as more carbohydrates.
- Reduce coffee and caffeine. Simply stated, caffeine increases insulin release.
- Eat adequate protein and healthy fats. Hormone stimulation requires proteins and fats. We need both to maintain a healthy balance.

Choose one of the bullets above to focus on this week. Stick to this one small step every day. It will soon become a habit.

12 www.cdc.gov/healthyschools/obesity/facts.htm

DIGESTIVE TIP CHECK IN: Real foods bring needed nutrients to our digestive systems. Processed foods and stress impair and deplete nutrients. Get Real suggests these nutrients because they are necessary for a healthy, vital system. Healthy digestion creates a healthy body.

DAY 5: AN HONEST PERSPECTIVE

As you have seen, we like to take a small step approach to making these lifestyle changes for your family. When we personally started this process, we didn't realize how much sugar was hiding in the products we were regularly choosing. Sugar was adding up fast. Below is a review of a pretty common food journal, we think you will be amazed at all the sugar lurking around.

FOOD JOUNAL: Elementary School Child

BREAKFAST		LUNCH		DINNER	
Danimals yogurt	8G SUGAR	Lunchable	30G SUGAR	Chicken nuggets	
Little bites	25G SUGAR	Fruit roll-up	7G SUGAR	Macaroni and	6G SUGAR
		Cheese		cheese	
				2 packaged cookies	18G SUGAR
				Small Gatorade®	20G SUGAR

TOTAL SUGAR/DAY: 114 G = **28.5 TEASPOONS**
RECOMMENDED: FOR KIDS AT THIS AGE IS NO MORE THAN 3 - 4 TEASPOONS PER DAY

FOOD JOUNAL: Adolescent Child

BREAKFAST		LUNCH		DINNER	
2 servings of cereal	20G SUGAR	Sandwich	4G SUGAR	Chicken breast in	
Milk	12G SUGAR	Chips		marinade	6G SUGAR
		Skittles (small bag)	10G SUGAR	Pasta and broccoli	
		Small Gatorade®	20G SUGAR	with sauce	9G SUGAR
				Ice cream sandwich	21G SUGAR
		SNACK			
		Clif® bar	22G SUGAR		

TOTAL SUGAR/DAY: 112 G = **28 TEASPOONS**
RECOMMENDED: 6 TEASPOONS OR LESS FOR GIRLS, 9 TEASPOONS OR LESS FOR BOYS

As we shift focus on an entire day, the point here is to recognize how quickly 'just a little' adds up to be a whole lot. Let's shift forward with some honest awareness. There will be no changes today, it will simply be a review of the total sugar we consume each day.

One day, I simply explained to my family what sugar does to their bodies, and all the places it was hiding. Then as a family we came up with realistic goals for the amount of sugar that would be allowed in a day. For us it was four things containing sugar, excluding fruit. This sounds like a lot, right? But when we really looked at our daily sugar intake, we realized it was so much more than that. - Amy

Once I started to notice my addiction to sugar and my energy shifts as I changed my diet, I also noticed it in my boys. This was a baby step process. We focused on one thing at a time. I started by trying to get the sugar out of breakfast and then slowly moved my way into the other meals. We started to cut out daily dessert and have it on weekends only. I also spoke to them about reading labels and asked them to notice if they feel any different when they ate less sugar. My goal for my kids is to bring awareness into their minds, this is an invaluable tool as they grow independent. - Mary

 Evaluate the food journal from each member of your family. Total the amount of grams of sugar consumed.

Day 6: CREATING HEALTHY HABITS

As children grow, we want to support their needs. We also know that their lives can be a little overwhelming so we are going to make recommendations than can happen with ease. As you choose to transition away from processed and high-sugar items, remember to keep it slow, be gentle and go easy on yourself—and them! Even in our own houses, sugar occasionally sneaks itself back in. So this is one chapter in particular we suggest revisiting together again and again.

No matter their age or stage, there's one constant: Change should be gradual. Sugar is a hot-button topic with children and adolescents. Let's focus on ways to include healthful foods and reduce sugar.

This next step is up to you. Choose one of the processed food/high sugar item from your child's day and transition it to a healthier form.

Example: If your child always has chips after school, serve some homemade popcorn instead (can be made ahead of time).

If you're used to chocolate milk in the mornings, measure out the serving and add a little less each week.

You choose what will be the best transition in your household. Remember, it doesn't have to be elaborate, it could be as simple as an apple with cinnamon.

> ## CREATING HEALTHY HABITS
> FIRST, LET'S ACKNOWLEDGE ALL THE HEALTHY SHIFTS YOU HAVE INCORPORATED.
> - ☑ SHIFTING FROM SODA/JUICES TO WATER.
> - ☑ STARTED TO LOWER OR ELIMINATE SUGAR INTAKE AT BREAKFAST.
> - ☑ STARTED TO INCREASE HEALTHY FATS.
>
> LET US REMIND YOU THAT THIS IS REMARKABLE.

Sugar is everywhere and patience is required for this process. Spend some time explaining this transition to your kids. Ask them questions. Let them make choices along the way.

ADOLESCENTS

"Energy nutrient needs are greater during adolescence than during any other time in life (except pregnancy and lactation)."[13]

TEEN DIET	HOME SOLUTIONS
High in sweets	Increase healthy options – keep junk food to a minimum
High in refined/processed foods	Increase complex carbohydrates, protein and healthy fats
High in fast food	Minimize take-out as a family
Soda consumption	Increase water intake as a family

Increased hormones and physical growth are hallmarks of adolescence. A balanced diet that's low in sugar and processed foods is the best support. Good nutrition will support healthy skin, healthy teeth (don't forget to floss) and balanced hormones. As always, hydrate with water.

At some point, our kids will go out and make their own choices. We want them to have these experiences to grow and learn. Stick to the 'Home Solutions' (above to the right) and that will keep more nutrient dense choices in their diet.

Today's teen has a lot of stress and a busy schedule. They need nutrients, patience, hugs and a little extra love. We highly recommend not hounding your teens about what they are snacking on away from home; let it be.

DAY 7: CELEBRATING CHANGE

Notice any physical or mental shifts that you've felt from these transitions. Recognizing the impact of these changes is great motivation to continue on this journey. Continue to notice how you feel when you add healthy, nourishing, real food and lower processed foods.

---

13 Whitney, E. and Rolfes, S. Understanding Nutrition. Boston: Wadsworth Learning, 2008. (560)

Start to choose healthier snacks.

A FEW OPTIONS

Apple sami (see recipe page 135)

Celery with nut butter

Cheese stick

Cottage cheese with berries and cinnamon

Crackers, peanut butter, mini chocolate chips and berries

Healthy bread or wrap with smashed avocado or nut butter

Healthy trail mix (nuts, dried fruit, coconut chips)

homemade potato skins

Jerky

Oat bars

Pick your fruit in the produce section

Plain yogurt with berries

Popcorn

Sliced apple with nut butter

Smoothie

Thin rice cake with nut butter

Vegetables and hummus

Try this healthier cookie recipe for an after-school snack.

CHOCOLATE COOKIES

INGREDIENTS: organic peanut butter, honey, sugar, egg, cocoa powder, chocolate chips, sea salt

1 cup	organic peanut butter	Blend all ingredients together. Place on baking stone or parchment lined cookie sheet.
¼ cup	honey	
¼ cup	sugar	Bake at 350 for 16 - 18 minutes. Let sit for 5 minutes prior to serving.
1	egg	
½ teaspoon	vanilla	
2-3 tablespoons	cocoa powder	OPTIONAL ADD IN: 1/4 cup dark chocolate chips
¼ teaspoon	sea salt	

CHECK IN: HOW IS YOUR HOUSEHOLD DOING WITH WATER INTAKE?

Are you drinking ½ your weight in ounces daily yet?
Still drinking soda, energy drinks and lattes?
- Start to decrease the size you order.

Wake up to a cup of coffee?
- Have a glass of water first.
- Choose one day to only drink water and herbal tea.

Week 6: LUNCHES

It takes some planning and prep work to change up a lunch routine—not only for ourselves, but also for our families. Mornings are busy, and it's difficult to break habits that save time and headspace. We're here to tell you that, with the right plan, Get Real lunches can actually be the easiest transition you tackle. Here's why: Once it's settled, there's no more guesswork.

Bringing a lunch prepared at home following our guidelines ensures you and your family will feel nourished and satisfied. A balanced lunch with nutrient-dense choices provides slow burning energy and fewer cravings throughout the day.

We will guide you through this transition with some quick and easy ideas that require a short amount of prep time in the morning. In addition, each day we will explain why commonly chosen lunch items are poor choices, while sharing healthy alternatives.

GET REAL REMINDER: This is a transition and it will take patience and time. Your family's lunches will not be completely transformed within a week. However, after this week you will be equipped with the knowledge to lead you in the right direction.

Sugar Love - One of the most common protests we hear from our clients is that they feel like it is "unloving" to stop sending a sweet treat to school with their children. Obviously, that's not true; but mindsets are powerful. So we've included a few ideas to let your loved ones know you're thinking of them during those long school days without the sugar rush. Remember, a little planning goes a long way.

- Make a note: Write a joke, or simply, "I love you." Let them know about something you've planned for later, for example: "Want to go to the park after school?"
- Stickers: The dollar store is full of stickers that you can put in fun places in a lunchbox or on a brown bag.
- Cut sandwiches into shapes: There are many different types of cookie cutters available online and in the grocery shop, and they're not just seasonal anymore.
- Silly straws: Keep these stashed and you never know when they will appear in a lunch box. Note: The straw is for water, of course!
- Toothpicks: Kids love eating mini kabobs!

You get the idea be creative and have fun!

Day 1: WHAT'S INSIDE (OR OUTSIDE) YOUR LUNCH BOX?

What does lunch look like to you and your family? Today, we'll be examining the mid-day meal in close detail and searching for balance. Here are some questions to start considering:

- How often do you eat lunch out?
- How often do your kids purchase lunch from the cafeteria?
- How much money are you spending on eating out at lunch?

ASK YOURSELF A FEW QUESTIONS IF YOU'RE ALREADY PACKING LUNCHES

- How many prepared foods do you and your family consume for lunch?
- What are you drinking with lunch?
- How much sugar is hiding in the lunchtime meal?
- How do you feel two hours after you eat your lunch?

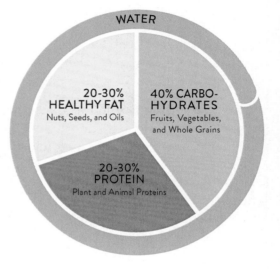

Balance is key during lunch. A balanced lunch will carry us through the day, preventing the need for that two o'clock coffee break or chocolate run.

Get Real lunches are prepared and packed at home. Packing a lunch at home has three enormous benefits

1. **Quality:** At home, you're more likely to choose real food.

2. **Time Saving:** Even though it might seem like a hassle to pack, you really do save time. When you pack lunch, you won't be stuck standing in line.

3. **Cost Effective:** All those lunches out add up. Not only will packing a balanced lunch save money, but it will ensure balance.

What's hiding inside prepared foods anyway? Let's take a closer look at the long list of ingredients inside a popular prepared food item, as compared with a Get Real alternative—that even has dark chocolate in it!

HOMEMADE VS. STORE BOUGHT

GET REAL's Lunchable

Nitrate free ham or turkey
Flat bread: whole wheat flour, unbleached wheat flour, filtered water, oat fiber, citric acid, yeast, sea salt, baking soda, cultured wheat.
Mustard: apple cider vinegar, water, mustard seed, sea salt, turmeric, paprika
Apple
Raw nuts
Piece of dark chocolate (cocoa beans, cane sugar, cocoa butter, ground vanilla bean)
Water

Lunchables

wild cherry water beverage with other natural flavor – water, high fructose corn syrup, citric acid, sucralose (Splenda® brand sweetener), natural flavor. bologna made with chicken & pork – mechanically separated chicken, water, pork, corn syrup, modified food starch, contains less than 2% of salt, potassium lactate, sodium phosphates, sodium diacetate, sodium ascorbate, flavor, sodium nitrite, extractives of paprika, potassium phosphate, sugar, potassium chloride. pasteurized prepared american cheese product – milk, whey, milk protein concentrate, milkfat, sodium citrate, contains less than 2% of salt, lactic acid, sorbic acid as a preservative, oleoresin paprika (color), annatto (color), enzymes, cheese culture, with starch added for slice separation. contains: milk. candy bar – corn syrup, sugar, ground roasted peanuts, hydrogenated palm kernel oil, cocoa, molasses, and less than 1% of whey (from milk), confectioner's corn flakes, nonfat milk, salt, lactic acid esters, soy lecithin, soybean oil, cornstarch, artificial flavors, tbhq and citric acid (added to preserve freshness), yellow 5, red 40. contains: peanut, milk, soy. crackers – unbleached enriched flour (wheat flour, niacin, reduced iron, thiamine mononitrate [vitamin B1], riboflavin [vitamin B2], folic acid), whole grain wheat flour, soybean oil, sugar, partially hydrogenated cottonseed oil, salt, leavening (baking soda and/or calcium phosphate), whey (from milk), soy lecithin, natural flavor.

Day 2: LET'S TALK LUNCH MEATS

The majority of meats in the deli case are cured with chemicals and preserved with artificial colors and flavors. The nitrates and use of high heat have also been found to be carcinogenic. Many types of meats contain undesired "fillers" or "meat glue." Let's not forget about all the antibiotics and hormones that are used in the growth of the animals or the pesticides used in the foods the animals ate. Many of these lunch meats will be labeled as 'natural,' but be advised to look deeper than that.

GET REAL APPROVED LUNCH MEATS ARE:

- Organic is best, but as long as the below bullets are in place, it is okay to skip organic and save some money
- Uncured meat has not been pre-served by smoking, salting or drying
- No nitrates and no nitrates added – both of these terms must be on the label[14]
- 100 % meat, which will ensure you don't get any fillers
- Ingredients should not list MSG, high fructose corn syrup or artificial colors/flavors.

LUNCH MEAT

RECOMENDED	VS.	STORE BOUGHT
GET REAL's Recommendation		**Processed Lunch Meat**
Organic pork, water. contains less than 2% of the following: sea salt, organic honey, organic cane sugar, celery powder		Ham, water, salt, contains less than 2% of sugar, sodium phosphates, sodium diacetate, sodium propionate, sodium benzoate, sodium ascorbate, sodium nitrate, soy lecithin

Processed meats also include nuggets, hot dogs, pepperoni, rotisserie chicken, sausage, bacon and jerky.

Day 3: CAFETERIA FOODS

The school cafeteria used to be a lot less healthy than it is today. Schools are doing some positive things to make meals more nutritious for their students, with support from advocates and the government. Recently, the old food pyramid was revised to include a model with more fruits and veggies that schools are now following as they plan their meals. Many states are passing regulations that have made their school cafeterias healthier, including adding more fresh fruit and vegetable options for kids who buy lunch, and even keeping sweets out of the classroom.

While many school cafeterias aren't the Jell-o and junk-laden minefields they once were, it's still always better to pack. Here's why: To keep the cost down, cafeteria foods are commonly prepared with hydrogenated oils, added sugar, high sodium and plenty of preservatives. In addition, you have less control over the quality of ingredients. Start to look at your child's school lunch menu, go to the website to see the actual ingredients that are being used. Many school cafeterias still don't have balanced options, are low fat, high carb and lacking in vegetables.

Again we would like to remind you food made from home is one of the easiest ways to guarantee quality as well as helping you save money. So we'd like to challenge you to start packing your kids' lunches just a few days a week.

---

14 One way that marketing has been very successful in tricking the consumer is by saying no nitrates added. This means the packing company has not added nitrates, however the food producer itself has used nitrates. Both must be on the label to ensure a nitrate free product.

Choice A:
- *If your child usually buys school lunch, plan to pack a lunch for them tomorrow.*
- *If you eat out everyday, plan to take a lunch to work.*

Don't worry about the contents of your lunch boxes yet, just get used to preparing and bringing a lunch from home.

Choice B: *If you usually pack a lunch that has mostly processed foods, replace one of the processed foods with another Get Real lunch replacement item or a piece of fruit. (See page 111 for some wholesome lunch ideas.)*

Day 4: TRANSITION TIPS & LUNCHBOX REBELLION

We have begun the transition to healthier lunches ... it's not always easy! Some kids may just rebel when they get a lunch box rather than carte blanch at the cafeteria. Anticipate their rebellion early by involving them in the transition and getting them excited about new options.

Today, we're going grocery shopping! Take your kids to the grocery store along with you, with the specific task to work just on lunches. So if you have to pick up dinner items or other staples, save that for another day. Today it's about focusing on lunch. Give each child a basket with the goal to fill it with the following:

- One protein
- One item from produce
- One packaged item

This is a great step to allow the kids to choose on their own. You may be surprised what they choose. Eventually, you will transition the one packaged item to a healthier option, but for now, let's keep something a little familiar in the lunch box.

My kids are not big fans of the store and a little older, which means they were set in their ways. So I started to transition the sandwiches first. The only thing that changed was the bread and the meat. Once balance was achieved, we focused on removing the chips. The first step was to have them every other day and we slowly weaned off chips altogether. Occasionally, I throw in a piece of dark chocolate as a treat, just to keep things interesting. (Why dark chocolate? Simply because it has less sugar.) I continue to pack homemade items, such as protein muffins, homemade granola bars and protein balls to fuel the kids before after school practice.—Mary

Look at your lunches. Choose the first transition item or find time for that family trip to the store.

Day 5: BREAD

"But, I buy whole wheat ..."

Take a minute to read the label on the breads you have in your house. You will notice there are several ingredients and a lot of processing that goes on to get bread to this soft, fluffy bread that has a long shelf life. We are not against carbohydrates our bodies need them. What we are against is extreme processing. Take a look at the bread labels below and let this be a guide as you begin to transition to a better bread choice. Regardless of what type of bread you are eating, most likely there is room for better quality choice.

BREAD TRANSITIONS

OVERALL REMINDER: The number one rule when buying bread is to always look for simple ingredients. In addition to the chart below, see our label review in the Q&A section 90.

BETTER CHOICES

Flat Bread

Unbleached wheat flour, filtered water, oat fiber, citric acid, yeast, sea salt, baking soda

Sprouted Bread

Organic sprouted wheat, filtered water, organic sprouted barley, organic sprouted millet, organic malted barley, organic sprouted lentils, organic sprouted soybeans, organic sprouted spelt, fresh yeast, organic wheat gluten, sea salt

Sourdough

100% Whole wheat flour, sea salt, water

White Bread

Enriched flour, wheat flour, malted barley flour, niacin, reduced iron, thiamine mononitrate, riboflavin, non fat milk, folic acid, water, high fructose corn syrup, yeast, wheat gluten, soybean oil, salt, butter, calcium carbonate, calcium sulfate

Whole Wheat Bread

Unbleached enriched flour, water, honey, sugar, wheat gluten, whole wheat flour, rye flour, wheat bran, yeast, soy, soy flour, soybean oil, monoglycerides, enzymes, ascorbic acid, cultured wheat flour, vinegar, calcium sulfate, monocalcium phosphate, soy lecithin, calcium carbonate

Gluten Free Bread

Water, potato extract, non GMO canola oil, rice starch, rice flour, evaporated cane syrup, inulin, bamboo fiber, honey, sea salt, molasses, egg whites, corn meal, sunflower oil, flax seed, millet, yeast, xanthan gum, distilled vinegar, natural enzyme

Remember, this is a transition. We aren't asking you to never eat another sandwich or hamburger. Just begin to notice. Try some of our breadless options and see how you feel.

Day 6: CHIPS

"What? No chips with lunch?"

Chips are a crunchy, salty snack many of us associate with a "balanced" lunch. Unfortunately, chips offer absolutely no nutrients. They're one of the biggest culprits when it comes to weight gain and most are highly processed.

Let's start with some label review. *INGREDIENTS: Spice, natural and artificial flavor, sodium citrate, disodium inosinate, and, disodium guanylate, nonfat milk solids, sugar, dextrose, malic acid, sodium caseinate, sodium acetate, artificial color (includes , red 40, blue 1, yellow 5), buttermilk solids, salt, tomato powder, partially hydrogenated soybean oil, corn syrup solids, corn starch, whey, onion powder, garlic powder, monosodium glutamate, cheddar cheese (cultured milk, salt, enzymes), corn, vegetable oil (contains one or more of the following: corn, soybean, sunflower oil)*

This a real label for a very common brand of chips. They are full of artificial colors, corn syrup, MSG, hydrogenated oils and so much more.

Some chip brands are beginning to be prepared with coconut oil and include less ingredients, and for a treat these are the better option. Please remember: While they are a better option, they still contain no nutrients, add to weight gain and are processed. These are a better option for an occasional snack.

Here are some delicious packed lunch ideas that include Get Real bread options and all the accompaniments.

- Flat wrap with leftover grilled chicken, romaine, white cheese, canteen of soup, nuts and chocolate.
- Sprouted bread with nut butter and honey, freeze dried strawberries, orange slices, and turkey jerky.
- Kid tip: This sandwich is perfectly bite-sized when cut into a cute shape using an old cookie cutter.
- Make your own pizza on flatbread with turkey pepperoni (no nitrates or nitrates added), and freshly grated mozzarella (sauce is optional). Add seasonal fruit, and granola bar for the crunch.
- Kid tip: Kids love to have their toppings in separate containers or a lunchtime bento box to prepare on their own.

Transition Steps:

Step 1 If you eat chips more than once a day, then start with having them just at lunch. (If you only have chips with lunch, skip to step 2.) Work with this concept for two weeks.

Step 2 Start to have chips only a few times a week, maybe every other day. Start to transition to those brands prepared with the least ingredients and cooked in healthy oil. Work with this concept for two weeks.

Step 3 Only have a healthier version of chips on occasion.

Day 7: ADD VEGGIES ONE AT A TIME

We realize that not all kids (and adults) are going to sit down and eat a salad with each meal. It can also be a little overwhelming during the transition to offer more than one type of vegetable at mealtime. The concept of separating veggies works especially well for those that are more resistant.

One example we've all probably tried is raw veggies and a dipping sauce. If your go-to is to always use baby carrots, start to introduce another vegetable this week. We like sliced cucumbers, or even celery for kids. For the adults, try some baby bells.

For the dipping sauce, use whatever works right now. If ranch dressing is all that will help your children eat some vegetables with lunch, then that's ok. This is a transition. You will find healthier options in our recipe section when you're ready to jump ahead.

As you continue to pack lunches this week start to add a vegetable.

Please know that this vegetable may come home everyday, but eventually it will be tried, and then it will be enjoyed. Your kids will come home and say, "Everyone else eats chips" or "Why do I have to be healthy?"

We all know that there are no nutrients in processed foods. This is a great time to bring this up to your child, and ask them to recognize how processed food makes them feel. Continuing to educate your kids will enable and empower them to be their healthiest, strongest and brightest.

If your child is especially resistant, give him or her some freedom in choosing. Continue to take your resistant child to the store and walk around the produce section. Play around with some options over the weekend to see which foods they will like.

Buy a lunch container that has separate compartments. These are sometimes called bento lunch boxes. The younger kids love to fill up the sections with you in the morning. This is a way to keep the lunch transition light and fun.

Get Real Lunch Recipes & Ideas

This list includes nutritious, balanced lunch options for adults and children that are incredibly simple to put together. They are packed with Real foods and are high on protein and veggies, low on carbs and sugar. We've included some delicious grownup options and some kid-pleasing lunchbox ideas, too. These lunches may feel very different from the lunches that you and your family are accustomed to eating. So please, take it slow.

For lunch recipes that require a few more steps, page 111. We've included our favorite salads, salad dressings and a few different types of quinoa bowl and soup recipes there for when you're feeling adventurous.

 Start transitioning to these options slowly. Find one lunch idea that sounds good for you, and one your children might enjoy. Start with that option one day a week until you're ready to try another. Take this slow, and enjoy the process!

ONE WEEK OF TRANSITIONAL BROWN BAG LUNCHES

- Peanut butter and honey on bread of choice, trail mix, sliced oranges
- Turkey jerky, sliced cheese, carrots, pretzels and a homemade dipping sauce
- Leftover soup in a canteen, trail mix
- Taco salad: romaine, cheese, leftover beef taco meat, tomatoes, avocado
- Taco roll up: tortilla with taco meat, cheese, dipping salsa, greens optional
- Make your own flatbread pizza with piece of fruit
- Make your own lunchable with Get Real approved meat

ONE WEEK OF CLEAN BROWN BAG LUNCHES

- Chicken salad with avocado over greens and seasonal fruit (Not ready for greens... Choose a healthier bread option)
- Flatbread with turkey, spinach, hummus, kalamata olives and seasonal fruit
- Quinoa salad with chopped nuts or seeds and seasonal fruit
- Shredded slaw with chicken
- Brown rice bowl with vegetables, avocado and pumpkin seeds (Option for other nut/protein)
- Chopped kale salad with apples, walnuts and half a sweet potato
- Bento box: hard boiled egg, raw veggies with guacamole and seasonal fruit

Week 7: REFLECTIONS

"As a man thinks so is he" Proverbs 23:7

This week, we'll be taking a break from food to focus on something a little different but no less integral to our health: our thoughts, words and actions. At Get Real, we believe that to live in complete health, we must address the power of our words and thoughts in relation to our health. There's a true scientific link[15] between stress levels and hormone balance, and studies that show positive thoughts influence healthier outcomes. However, this week is also about paying attention to your family's emotional wellbeing, checking in, and creating space for positive affirmation and quiet reflection.

Day 1: THE SPOKEN WORD

Our words are powerful, there is no question about this. But are we using them correctly? So often the words we use can become automatic, just like the mindless choices we make at snack time. It makes perfect sense that there is science to back the power of self-talk to affect outcomes.

Can you remember a time when you were deeply hurt by the words used by someone you loved, or even someone you barely knew? Now think back to a time when you felt affirmed by positive words from someone in your life. The power of our words strikes deep, and lasts long after they are spoken.

Today take a minute to listen to the "talk" that's going on in your house. Is it encouraging? As a family, are you building each other up or tearing each other down?

Give yourself some room. We understand that life has its demands. Between work, school, and all that's in-between, our family time can become a meeting of really tired people at the end of a long day.

> *Something we do at our house is called "Take 10." Everyone understands that it's necessary to regroup in order to be kind. So after school our kids take 10 minutes to themselves in their own rooms to wind down and just be. No phones, TV, or gaming allowed. Just peace and quiet. This allows them the time to regroup and be ready to treat each other the way we would want to be treated. Mom and Dad also take 10 after work. (Sometimes we may need to take 30!) - Amy*

Day 2: THE UNSPOKEN WORDS

It's really true that we have to start with ourselves. Today think about the thoughts that aren't spoken. What kind of thoughts run through your head when you're driving, exercising or even listening to other people? We don't even notice how many negative thoughts stream through our minds on a consistent basis. These thoughts do matter. What is the underlying message you're speaking to yourself all day?

Through our work with our own clients, we've noticed that negative thoughts often revolve around two things: body image and time management. Do you find yourself thinking about all the things you can't get done in a day's time? Or wishing you looked different, focusing on what you don't like about your body?

Today, allow yourself to recognize these negative thought patterns and then take a moment to find the truth in your thoughts. There is nothing wrong with recognizing the need to be in better health, but with the same thought we need to recognize all the many functions that our bodies perform for us on a daily basis that we often take for granted.

Our overall goal is health, acceptance and love of self and others.

Negative thought: I've completely failed my family in this transition to a real foods plan.

Truth: This transition is a work in progress. My family's water consumption is up quite a bit and that's a win.

I had to decide that getting a healthy dinner in during the weeknights would take priority over my children's socks matching. This sounds funny but anyone with a big family knows that keeping matching socks on everyone is a chore. I realized I had enough time in my day, but I just chose to use it on the things that would have a long-term effect on my children's health. - Amy

My house isn't perfect, and you'll probably find dishes in my sink if you come over unannounced. But as my kids grew older, they were given more responsibilities. For example, we taught our boys how to do their own laundry! They have all taken ownership of this and we usually call it the "laundry train" to get it moving through the weekend. At times, my husband and I will help them. But overall they wash and organize their clothes on their own. This gave the parents a little more time to get a healthy dinner on the table or to run out to the store for some fresh foods. - Mary

Day 3: AFFIRMATIONS

Today, we're going to suggest affirmations to incorporate into your routine. Affirmations are positive, true statements that we intentionally choose to focus on. We have a choice to connect to a negative thought that's most likely based on fear, or we can choose to connect to a positive thought that's connected with the truth. The first step is to recognize these negative thoughts. Our second step is to create a new path for our thoughts. The third—and truly powerful step for you and your family—is to speak these new positive thoughts aloud in the form of affirmations.

Teachers have creative and effective ways to build positive environments in their classrooms and often use the trick of affirmations to keep their students focused, feeling confident and to preserve a positive social environment. In fact, the Get Real affirmations below were first introduced by a preschool teacher.

GET REAL AFFIRMATIONS

- I am brave, bold and courageous.
- I am not fearful, but I am powerful, loving and have a sound mind.
- I am quick, sharp and bright.

We realize that these exact affirmations may not work for you, but you get the idea: take time to think of a few positives today.

Try speaking this affirmation at dinner with your family. If speaking it out loud doesn't work well, another option is to write it down. Have each person in your family write down a positive statement and place it in a bowl in the center of the table. You can read each other's out loud, or silently.

When my kids were a lot younger, one of them was motivated by negative attention. I read of an idea to have an "I saw that" jar. Rather than consistently giving attention during those negative moments, I would recognize when they were being extra nice in some way. The jar was filled with special privileges such as extra screen time, playing their favorite board game and/or some other activity we could do together. This lasted a few months and helped transition my son away from that negative motivation he was always seeking. - Mary

Day 4: COMPLIMENT

Take time today to write one positive thing about each member in your household, and post it somewhere they will see it. We have included a few ideas here, or you can do your own with sticky notes.

Just watch. When we speak kind words to each other, we set the stage for positive change. It means recognizing that person and showing that you care.

GET REAL PERSONAL AFFIRMATIONS

- You are kind.
- You are an amazing friend.
- You are a loyal employee.
- You are such a help around the house.

When we brought our oldest child home from the hospital, like most new parents we had no idea what to do. Apparently, lying on the bed watching my husband swaddle our daughter in her blanket, I said to him, "You are the best dad ever." I don't remember this but years later my husband has told me the words I spoke to him in that moment created a new reality for him. He knew he was two days into being a father and that I had grown up with an amazing father, but the fact that I believed in him made him want to be the best dad he could be. Our words are powerful! - Amy

Day 5: SURVIVAL GOALS

Are you just surviving? We've all been at the point where just getting through the day is all we can set out to do. And let's Get Real, sometimes that's okay. Today, take time to make a list of places where you're thriving and places you're surviving. Now pick one place on your list that has changed for the better in the last six months and take time to appreciate it.

Now pick another place where you're surviving and let's set some goals to help change that. We believe in finding real life answers. The steps we take in change can be small, but we will feel benefit even from the most subtle changes if they're right.

Day 6: RANDOM ACTS OF KINDNESS

When we sit and think of acts of kindness, we're likely to come up with plenty of ideas. Often, we get these ideas and then forget all about them. What if you had impulses to do something kind, and acted on them?

What if you acted on them and had no expectation for something in return?

It's like that concept, "pay it forward," where one act of kindness leads to another and it just keeps building. Kindness is a choice we have in this beautiful life. Our actions are extremely powerful. These simple acts can change the course of a person's day.

Today the focus is on helping others, when we know there is nothing they can give back. Some habits come natural and some we have to train ourselves to do. Training ourselves and our kids to look for opportunities to help others is a great place to start, and always rewarding. Think back to a time when someone went out of their way to be kind to you. Write it down, and share the memory with your family. Brainstorm acts of kindness you can each set out to do.

EXAMPLES OF SIMPLE ACTS OF KINDNESS

- Wait to hold the door for someone.
- Pick up trash without it being an organized event.
- Simply notice something about someone and take time to compliment it.
- Once you perform this gesture, move forward and don't look back. Let it be.

> *As our kids entered grade school they would occasionally feel reluctant to go to school. So we created something called "Secret Mission." As I would drop them off, I would tell them something to do that day as their Secret Mission. It would be something simple like talk to someone at school you have never spoke to before, or look for the opportunity to say something nice to a teacher or tell the janitor thank you.*
>
> *Secret Mission became a favorite activity at our house. This is why: It gave our kids purpose, and it shifted their mindsets from thinking about themselves to thinking of others. Anytime any of us look to encourage and find good in others we can't help but feel good. - Amy*

Day 7: THE POWER OF PERSPECTIVE
Our thoughts inform our perspective.

Often times we see things in a certain way and that creates a specific viewpoint. Sometimes it's helpful to take a step back and look at a situation from a different angle. This allows us to not only see things a little different, but it also gives us the ability to zoom out and maybe see the whole, rather than just a part.

It is common to play a continuous narrative in certain situations that is informed by worry or fear. As we continue to follow these thought patterns of worry, we create undue stress. A stressful mind creates a stressful body. Stress has a huge impact on our hormone levels, our digestive function, the balance of our system and can greatly impact inflammation.

Sometimes the best way to deal with perspective is to take a moment to simply pause. Sit quietly and focus on some breathing exercises, enjoy a quiet walk in nature, do an enjoyable activity that requires focused attention, perform an act of kindness, journal, go to a yoga class, etc. We need to train ourselves to stop, pause and find a way to link to the present moment.

 Spend the day paying attention to these thought patterns. Find a renewed approach. Stop, listen and pause. See what happens.

Remember in Week 1, we touched on how much activity you and yours are getting? It's time to revisit this. Are you getting your heart rate up at least 5 days a week for 20 minutes of consistent activity? Can you touch your toes without discomfort or take the stairs and maintain a conversation? These simple suggestions may seem elementary but they are easy general markers for fitness. Want to know more? Check out our fitness topic in the Q&A section in the back of the book ("What is my target heart rate?" on page 96).

Week 8: TACKLING DINNER

In many households, the evening hours are extremely busy. Parents are getting home from work, kids often have activities and somewhere between it all we need to find a nourishing meal. Unfortunately, there simply aren't many places outside of the home that offer healthy meals for a family. Plus, the many benefits of eating real food prepared at home will always outweigh take out.

Before getting started on dinner, let's take a minute to reflect on how many changes we've already made together. Maybe your family has conquered breakfast or perhaps you're all drinking more water. Even if you've simply become more aware that change is happening, that's a big step. At this point, you may also be preparing your breakfasts and lunches at home, which means making the transition to preparing dinner at home is less daunting.

Remember the word transition. This is a transition and it does not have to be perfect! With that in mind, let's tackle dinner together. Over the next week we will begin to embrace bringing healthy options into our evenings.

See recipes starting on page 121 for menu ideas.

The Get Real POLITE PASS

The polite pass system helps take some of the tension out of dinner. Not only does Polite Pass give kids some "power," but it also makes it easier for reluctant adopters to try new recipes. Once they know they don't have to like everything, they might just be more open to new things.

Here's how it works:

- *Everyone is given the option to use two polite passes each week. (Adults included.)*
- *Polite passes don't roll over to the next week's meals.*
- *Post your menu for the week somewhere where everyone can see what is coming. This way, picky eaters can choose what they need to use their polite pass on.*
- *Polite pass can be declared after trying a meal and not liking it or prior to a meal.*
- *Once polite pass has been declared whoever is using their pass has to come up with their own meal. The parent is not to get up and prepare something else. The pass user can make a sandwich or eat leftovers.*

In my house pasta was a staple. As I started to transition away from serving pasta multiple times a week, I did not take it away, I simply made less and added a vegetable. Some nights I would mix the vegetables in with the pasta, some nights they would be separate. Once the kids were eating the vegetables, I started to transition the pasta out. Do my kids ever eat pasta? Yes, but it is infrequent and no longer a staple. - Mary

Day 1: MENU PLANNING

The key to making dinners fit into our schedule is preparation! If the ingredients aren't on hand, then takeout becomes the easy choice. We've included some simple steps to review today to begin preparations for Get Real dinner time. Just read these tips to start, then find the time to fit them into your schedule. That might not be today, and it's okay. Getting into a routine that includes looking ahead, meal planning and carving out time for the store will come.

1. Look at your calendar to get a plan for the week ahead. Plan your easiest meals on the busiest nights. (We have a list of easy meals waiting for you on the following pages.)

2. Make a menu (before you shop). Keep the meals simple. Save the meals that require a little more time for the weekend or a day when you can prep ahead. Refer to page 99 for meal plans that may work well for your family this week.

3. Go to the grocery store. The grocery store can be a fun and rewarding time, or it can be the place of the biggest struggles. We've all been taken down by an unruly toddler in a checkout line, or experienced the urge to eat the whole bag of chips while strolling through the aisles. Check out our tips on Day Four for managing this task.

4. It's okay to skip veggies this week! As you start the transition, don't worry about how many vegetables are being served. The first step is eating foods prepared in your kitchen. Once you get the hang of eating from home, you can work on including more vegetables.

5. Get some help with meal prep. If this week's budget allows, buy some prepped food for immediate use. Many produce sections now carry pre-cut veggies, diced onions, and peeled and cut fruit. Indulge in some while you get into the swing of things.

6. Post your menu. Having a plan takes away the daily guess work of what's for dinner for you, and your family members. Be sure to post your menu in a place where the whole family can see it. This will allow everyone to share in the transition and know what's coming.

We want to encourage you to just give it a try. Decide on a the amount of meals that you can realistically eat at home and go for it. Remember this is a transition!

 Choose what three meals you will prepare at home this week.

Day 2: MEAL PREP

You've already made a menu, planned for it and gone to the grocery store to stock up on ingredients. Today is about preparation. Look at your menu and ask yourself if there's anything you can do to prepare for the week ahead. Ideally, this day will fall on a weekend or a day that you have an extra hour or two to spend planning ahead.

MEAL PREPARATION TIPS

COOK GROUND MEAT
(or an extra protein choice.) This prep can be used for lunch or another evening meal. Use a simple spice or flavor so it can easily be used for a different meal.

INCLUDE LUNCH
While you're prepping for dinners, make extras for lunches too. Make a few salads and place them in separate containers ready to go. Could leftovers be tomorrow's lunch?

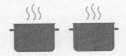

DOUBLE UP
Make a double batch of something that can freeze easily. Try our beef and vegetable soup on page 122. This is a huge time saver for a week or two ahead.

CHOP YOUR VEGETABLES
Place them in a separate container for each meal you plan to make. Have some frozen vegetable on hand as a time saver.

GET OUT THE CROCK POT
We know mornings are crazy, but a quick crock pot meal is so worth it for the time you save in the evening. Crock pots can be a wonderful way to prepare delicious Real Food. Check out our chicken pile on, orange chicken and crock pot ribs recipes on page 123.

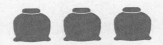

BUY STAPLE ITEMS IN BULK
Items such as brown rice, quinoa or frozen vegetables can be very helpful for a quick fix dinner. Some nights it's best to simplify, and use what you have.

GET OTHERS INVOLVED
Younger kids can help chop, if you supervise and help with safe knife skills. Bring your little children into the kitchen and catch up on the day while you're cooking. Teenagers can get dinner started. This can be as simple as turning the oven on or off. These extra hands can make a big difference.

TAKE IT SLOW
For some it's easier to plan the weekly menu and others work best within a 24-hour time frame rather than preparing for the entire week. For example, if you're making chicken for dinner, make extra for lunch. While you're cleaning up from dinner, pack your lunch for the next day. Before you go to bed, prepare anything you may need for breakfast.

Prepare and eat three meals at home this week.

Day 3: QUICK FIX OPTIONS

Some nights we get home and have a short time frame before we're out the door again. Check out a few of the quick fix options below to get through jams like these. Each quick fix recipe only takes 15-20 minutes to prepare. Once you get in the swing of eating from home, you'll find how rewarding it can be to get in some quality nourishment amid a hectic evening.

In order to be ready for quick fix options, note which options work best in your household and have those items available. Being prepared is a big factor when trying to maintain healthy choices.

Over the last few years of transitioning, I noticed that when things get really busy or when we've been traveling, even the kids start asking to just eat something simple at home. They recognize the difference in food quality and ease of eating at home. Take it slow and know the same will come to you over time. - Amy

GET REAL QUICK FIX DINNERS

Breakfast for Dinner

Make omelets with your favorite leftovers as fillers.

French toast is a kid favorite (recipe on page 110).

Serve soft boiled eggs over greens.

Stir Fry

Have some ground meat in the freezer or fridge ready to go.

Have some frozen vegetables in the freezer.

Prepare more than one batch of rice or quinoa early in the week, and keep extra in the fridge.

Burgers

Meals don't need to be fancy to be a hit.

Skip the buns and top with sauteed onions and quality pickles.

Skip the buns and top with salsa and guacamole.

Not ready to skip the bun? Try thin buns. Look for one with eight ingredients or less.

Quick Chili

Cook ground turkey, black beans, pepper, canned chopped tomato and your favorite seasoning. Chili doesn't have to take all day, this version can be ready in 15 minutes, and takes less than five minutes to throw together! Top with raw cheddar, sliced onions and some avocado or guacamole.

Chili wasn't a favorite for my kids, so I turned Chili night into soda night. Every once in awhile, when chili came to the table everyone got a soda. It worked like magic: Suddenly all the chili disappeared, too! - Amy

One Skillet Meals

Sauté chicken and vegetables with coconut oil. Load up the vegetables.

Beef and Broccoli (try our easy recipepage 121)

Lemon Chicken (kids love this recipe, page 127)

Easy Spaghetti

Add some ground meat and jarred sauce to your spaghetti.

A note about jarred sauce: *Read the label and look for added sugar. When reading your label, try to include only real food ingredients that you can pronounce. Or pick up the fresh stuff you find in the deli section at most supermarkets. It's okay to make a little pasta as your family is transitioning. Try to keep the serving size in check for the pasta and serve a vegetable that your kids will like along with it.*

Brown Rice or Quinoa Bowl

The options for filling your "bowl" are endless, satisfying and delicious. We have a few ideas in the lunch section try "Rainbow Quinoa or brown rice" on page 114 or see a list of bowl options in the index "Bowls" on page 139. You can set up a bar and have your family members make their own creations.

At a game or event all night?

Here are a few easy-to-pack and easy-to-eat meals:

Ham and Cheese Kabobs with fruit.

Clean Hot Pocket: Toast flat bread under the broiler, add pesto or marinara and top with mozzarella. You can add Canadian bacon, or grilled chicken- whatever veggies you have on hand and basically you made a clean hot pocket!

Greek Bowl: Blend tomato, cucumber, feta and red onion. Mix with quinoa.

Day 4: THE GROCERY STORE

"Our best and worst eating habits start at the grocery store. Food that's bought here gets moved into our homes. Food in our homes gets eaten."[16]

Buying groceries is expensive! Get Real shopping prioritizes spending based on the below list.

1. Quality oils take priority. Remember Week Four? As you transition to Real Foods, you'll be slowly stocking up on good quality oils and fats like olive oil, coconut oil, butter and nut butter. (See full list on page 45). These cost more, but are worth the investment.

2. A good source for meats and eggs. Remember that natural is often just a term used in marketing. When it comes to protein, choose organic if you can. If not, remember simply that eating meats prepared from home using clean seasonings and proper cooking technique is a big win.

3. Produce. While the Get Real plan does recommend organic or local produce in most instances, it's not always a mandate. At times, you can prioritize which products to buy organic and find the best quality you can afford for the other items. Check out page 91 to learn about the Clean 15 and the Dirty Dozen and work from this list to determine when to buy organic. We can't stress enough whatever produce you buy, wash it well. It's a win to be eating fresh produce, do remember that as you make your choices.

4. Packaged foods. If you're transitioning or just not ready to go all fresh yet, that is okay. But remember that just because a packaged food is labeled organic or gluten free, that doesn't mean it's a health food.

 Is there a certain processed food that is a staple in your house? If so, replace it with something else or buy it every other week instead.

Day 5: EATING OUT OPTIONS

Inevitably, we will have to eat out and want to eat out, too. Eating out is part of being in a community, and it can be a lot of fun. We're not opposed to dining out when the moment is right, so let's follow some Get Real tips to make the experience healthier.

1. Look to see if the restaurant has a 'healthy' option section or ask. This is often helpful and they will refine the meal to have a more appropriate serving. Ask your server, they can easily modify the meal and options for you.

2. Pass the Bread: Just say, "no thank you" and the server will remove your bread basket from the table.

---

16 Wansink, Brain. Slim by Design: Mindless Eating Solutions for Everyday Life. Harper Collins, 2014.

3. Appetizers: Appetizers can be skipped, unless you choose the item for your meal. Some restaurants may have a healthier appetizer, which would pair nicely with a soup or salad. Or, order a side salad as soon as your seat hits the seat. This works especially well when eating out with groups, because you don't become vulnerable to appetizers.

4. Soup: Broth-based soups can sometimes provide the healthiest choice. Add a side salad and you will have a healthy, satisfying and delicious meal.

5. Vegetables: Instead of ordering the rice or potato, order two vegetables to go with your protein.

6. Portion Control: Watch the size of the protein and grain on your plate; it's often enough to feed two. Remember it's easy to ask for a to-go box as soon as your meal comes and split your portion before you even begin to eat.

7. Wrap It: If you're not quite ready to give up your weekly burger or favorite chicken sandwich that's ok! Next time, lose the top bun and enjoy. Several places—even fast food places—will be happy to wrap your burger or sandwich in a lettuce wrap instead.

8. Water Instead of Soda: This not only has health benefits but also financial benefits. If everyone in a family of four drinks only water with a meal out, the bill will be 10-15 dollars cheaper. If you're still transitioning, order only one soda with no refills.

9. Choose Simply: Be aware of the sugars and oils hiding in restaurant meals. To make foods taste 'good,' restaurants often load them up with sugar and prepare them with hydrogenated oils. These two ingredients cause a lot of stress on our systems (review Weeks 4 & 5).

Day 6: COMPARISON

We often hear that it is expensive to eat healthy and we would like to take some time to compare dinner options. We also want to acknowledge that yes, your grocery bill will go up if you're preparing more dinners at home. But in the end, you save money because your restaurant bills will go down. In addition, you're adding quality, nutrient-rich foods into our home.

Budget Breakout

Take-out Meal for Family of 4:
4 Chicken Sandwich Combos

TOTAL COST: **$30 (average receipt)**

OR

Crock Pot Garlic Orange Chicken:

Chicken (2 drumsticks/person)	COST: $8.00
1 Orange	COST: $1.00
Garlic Clove	COST: $0.25
Rice	COST: $1.00
Tamari	COST: $0.75
Broccoli	COST: $3.00
TOTAL COST:	**$13.00**

Continue to notice the amount of time your household eats out. Recognize while your grocery bill may have increased your expenses at restaurants have decreased. Compare this shift in spending to your first week.

Eat Mindfully. Do not work while you eat. Instead, enjoy the company of a friend or enjoy your meal without distraction. Put your fork down in between each bite.

Day 7: FAMILY MEALS

Family meals can mean so much more than sitting down and eating together. Invite your kids and spouse into the entire process. Bringing family members into the dinner process gives them a voice. It also helps them see that there is always a healthier version.

A FEW IDEAS

- When making your menu for the week, ask each person in your family for one meal suggestion. You can always use Pinterest or another resource to find a healthier version of their requests.
- Have kids help out with meal prep. Bringing kids into the kitchen is so important! Let them see the variety of produce, let them chop, and eventually let them cook. We also love to let them clean up.
- If other members of your family are not quite on board consider making a few transitional meals, or just cleaning up some of their favorite recipes. Check out "OK Enchilada Casserole" on page 129.
- Sit down and eat the meal together. Take your time. Yes, we are busy and this most likely won't happen every night. But when it does, the experience is invaluable. Sitting around the table and enjoying time with family is a sharing and building experience.

Bonus Challenge: Eat two family meals together this week.

On weekends, my absolute favorite dinner is something grilled with a creative salad. My husband loves to grill and the kids are usually hanging out close by. Once the grill goes on at my house, it brings community and I love that time with family and friends. - Mary

WHAT ABOUT DESSERT?

While we don't recommend dessert on a daily basis, one of the great things about making healthy living a lifestyle is that on occasion, dessert is just fine. Go ahead and enjoy that pumpkin pie or birthday cake. Remember, this is a lifestyle transition. So it's best to enjoy everything in moderation.

Once you've cleared sugar from your diet on a daily basis, you may realize that the cookie or cake that once was so irresistible, doesn't taste so good. You also will find balance to know when to enjoy and when to back off. We are sure of this!

AFTER DINNER EATING

Sometimes busy schedules call for an early dinner. That might lead to hunger later on in the evening. Plus, adolescents who participate in sports can burn off an early dinner very quickly. We don't recommend eating right before bed or choosing a food that is high sugar or mostly carbohydrates, because this can affect sleep patterns.

GET REAL LATE-NIGHT SNACK IDEAS

- Smoothies. After dinner, try making them more like 'ice cream.' Use frozen fruit, protein powder and coconut milk.
- Trail mix. Add some dark chocolate to a homemade blend of nuts and apricots or raisins.
- Oatmeal cookies. (See page 136 for recipe.) They are easy to make a double batch and freeze.
- Another meal. Some evenings, leftover dinner is the best option.
- Homemade popcorn with coconut oil goes well with a movie.
- Rice cakes and nut butter topped with mini chocolate chips
- Cheese slices and turkey breast
- Granola, nut butter and honey all mixed together.
- Coconut bites. (See recipe on page 136.)
- Wraps. Grab leftover meat from dinner or quality lunch meat, a few slices of cheddar and healthy wraps.

By now, you and your family have celebrated many wins. Reading until the end of this book is itself a big win! You may have already drastically reduced your soda consumption, cut back on sugar, found some healthy and fun lunch ideas and enjoyed a family meal together while sharing positive words of encouragement and affirmation.

Over the next pages, you'll find all the tools you and your family need to carry on with the Get Real lifestyle transition. We've included two weeks of transitional meal plans and two weeks of cleaner meal plans for when you're ready. All of the corresponding recipes are included in the index of this book. Always remember that this is a lifestyle transition. Choose the plans and meals that feel best for you, your preferences, lifestyle and needs.

We challenge you to keep this book somewhere that you will return to it from time to time. After you've incorporated some of our small steps, revisit the pages and fine tune your lifestyle transition. Getting Real is a constant work in progress!

Get Real Q&A

We've noticed that many of our nutrition clients have asked many of the following questions as they embarked on their own Get Real transitions. When it comes to nutrition, we're up against so much conflicting, confusing and even misleading information. The following Q&A section is designed to clear up some of the common misconceptions and answer many of the questions we hear the most frequently.

Q: What is a balanced meal?

Carbohydrates, proteins and fats are macronutrients, which should be present and balanced in each meal. Water is also a key component of a balanced meal.

Drink one half your body weight (ounces of water) throughout the day.

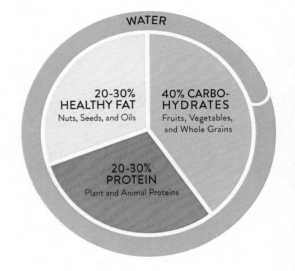

We have also mentioned that this is not a perfect ratio for everyone. Depending on activity, genetics, healing and other factors, we will need to shift this throughout our lives. This is where keeping a food journal is highly beneficial. We also recommend checking in with the mini-quiz on page 50 to see how the prior meal affected our cravings, energy and disposition.

Practicing awareness and listening to your body is essential here.

Many people have more carbohydrates in their diet with lower protein and healthy fats. On page 56, we discussed the cycle of cravings and hormone dysfunction a high carbohydrate diet can create. Including more fruits and vegetables also creates more balance due to the abundance of micronutrients (vitamins and minerals). These nutrients are essential and have many roles in our bodies.

Continue to enjoy our recipes and notice what feels best and balanced for you. Remove processed foods and sugar. Choose REAL FOOD!

Q: *How do I make sense of nutritional labels? Which labels mean something, and which ones are gimmicks?*

Here's our Get Real guide to understanding labels and outsmarting marketers while loading up on what's Real! Remember Get Real's recommendation is for you to eat food closest to its original source, but we also recognize the need to live within a budget. Being smart consumers helps us to understand where to spend our money and when marketing is getting the best of our dollar.

UNDERSTANDING LABELS
MEAT, EGGS AND DAIRY LABELS

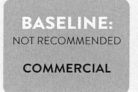

BASELINE:
NOT RECOMMENDED

COMMERCIAL

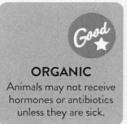

Good

ORGANIC
Animals may not receive hormones or antibiotics unless they are sick.

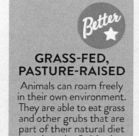

Better

GRASS-FED, PASTURE-RAISED
Animals can roam freely in their own environment. They are able to eat grass and other grubs that are part of their natural diet and can be finished.

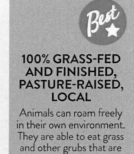

Best

100% GRASS-FED AND FINISHED, PASTURE-RAISED, LOCAL
Animals can roam freely in their own environment. They are able to eat grass and other grubs that are part of their natural diet.

MEAT, EGGS AND DAIRY LABELS

PASTURE-RAISED: Animals can roam freely in their own environment. They are able to eat grass and other grubs that are part of their natural diet.

ORGANIC: Animals may not receive hormones or antibiotics unless they are sick. They consume organic feed and have outdoor access. Animals are not necessarily grass-fed. Compliance is verified through third-party auditing.

NATURAL: This means minimally processed. Warning: This word is often used as a marketing ploy. All cuts are minimally processed by definition and free of flavorings and chemicals.

CAGE-FREE: Poultry is uncaged, mostly inside barns or warehouses, but they generally don't have access to the outdoors. There is no third-party auditing.

FREE RANGE: Poultry must have access to the outdoors 51 percent of the time. Other animals may not be in feedlots. There are no restrictions on what can be fed to the animals.

VEGETARIAN FED: This implies that the animal feed is free of animal bi-products. Chickens are not vegetarian so the label just serves to indicate the chicken is not eating their natural diet.

A NOTE ABOUT BUYING DAIRY: Dairy is a builder, so it should be treated like a meal, not a condiment or drink. Buy whole, organic milk. Skim and one percent milk are highly processed. If you want to dilute for taste, do so simply with water. Stay away from pre-sweetened milk products or yogurts.

UNDERSTANDING LABELS

SEAFOOD

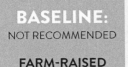

BASELINE:
NOT RECOMMENDED

FARM-RAISED

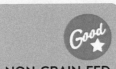

NON-GRAIN-FED

Fish are farmed "closer" to its natural diet & habitat.

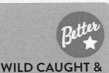

WILD CAUGHT & REALEASED

The fish may have lived in a fish farm before being returned to the wild and eventually caught.

WILD CAUGHT FISH

The fish was spawned, lived in & caught in the wild.

ALWAYS READ THE LABEL!
ALWAYS READ THE INGREDIENTS!

IN

Note size of servings.

Ingredients should be easily identified.

Package listed with no more than 5 or 6 ingredients.

AVOID

Artificial sweeteners (aspartame, sucralose, saccharin)

Artificial colors

Artificial flavors

Flavor enhancers (MSG, nitrates, maltodextrin, sodium benzoate)

Bad oils (hydrogenated, partially-hydrogenated, vegetable oils, canola, margarine)

High Fructose Corn Syrup

WHEN TO CHOOSE ORGANIC: If you need to choose, prioritize the "dirty dozen" first.

CLEAN FIFTEEN

Avocados
Sweet corn
Pineapples
Cabbage
Sweet peas, frozen
Onions
Asparagus
Mangos

Papayas
Kiwi
Eggplant
Honeydew melon
Grapefruit
Cantaloupe
Cauliflower

DIRTY DOZEN

Strawberries
Apples
Nectarines
Peaches
Celery
Grapes
Cherries

Spinach
Tomatoes
Sweet bell peppers
Cherry tomatoes
Cucumbers

SOURCE: The Environmental Working Group https://www.ewg.org/foodnews/

PRODUCE SKUS:

ORGANIC

 OR

CONVENTIONALLY GROWN

GENETICALLY MODIFIED - AVOID

GET REAL Q&A

Q: How should I navigate the grocery store in the most Real way?

From the moment we step into the store we are bombarded with unhealthy choices trying to sound like the perfect choice through clever marketing. We have all heard 'shop the perimeter' of the store, but even these sections have plenty of choices that are highly processed.

Helpful Tips:

1. **Don't go hungry:** We are more likely to choose items off our list if we're shopping hungry.

2. **Stick to the menu:** This is effective and a money saver. We like to organize our menu in categories to be efficient while shopping. It's also a big time saver.

3. **Read the Label:** If there are products that seem like a good choice, always read the label. Consider the value of nutrients. A simple question to ask yourself: Is this a healthy choice?

4. **Aisle Shopping:** There are some condiments, oils, paper goods, etc. that will continue to bring us down the aisle. Stick to tip number three when you're in the aisle, and read the ingredients.

Q: What is gluten?

Gluten is a protein found in grains (like wheat, rye, spelt, semolina, kamut and barley). Think of gluten as a 'glue.' It makes the dough sticky and gives bread its soft texture. The element of 'stickiness' is why it is used as a binding agent in many products. Gluten can be found in breads, crackers, baked goods, pasta, chips, pretzels and oats (through cross-contamination). Surprisingly, gluten is also found in alcohol, lunch meats, candy, dry roasted nuts, gravies, instant foods, processed meats/fish, sauces, vegan substitutes, soy sauce, salad dressing, marinades, bouillon cubes, fats used for frying, ice cream cones, thickener in ice cream, malted milk, mayonnaise, ovaltine and even vitamins.

Q: What are some other words and phrases for gluten that can be found on a food label?

Hydrolyzed vegetable protein, food starch, vegetable protein and natural flavors.

Q: Should I stop eating gluten?

Many of us have always eaten bread products, but in our busy lives we have also included more processed foods in our diet. Over time, the form of gluten has changed (through hybridization) and the current variation of the protein comes in a form that our body does not recognize, one that challenges us digestively. Pair this with the abundance of gluten products in our diet and our bodies come to a place where they cannot always handle its digestion. Consuming too much of this form of gluten can lead to inflammation, digestive imbalance and autoimmune conditions.

While it is best for some to avoid gluten altogether, it's important for others to lower their intake of these processed foods. There are also ways we can properly prepare grains to be more nutrient-dense and bring ease to our digestive process.

One more thing… if you are gluten free, continue to read the label. Many "gluten free" products are filled with sugars for the binding process. We stay true to our recommendation of choosing real foods first.

Q: **Is Carb a four-letter word?**

There is so much information out there pertaining to carbohydrates. Are they good? Bad? Will eating a banana make me fat? Let's sort through some basic information about carbohydrates to clear up some of these concerns.

Macronutrients consist of carbohydrates, proteins, fats and water. Carbohydrates provide fuel for the brain and are a quick source of energy for muscles. They also provide a good source of fiber, which is beneficial to the elimination process. Certain carbohydrates also feed the digestive system to help maintain a healthy gut (think greens).

We also hear the carbohydrates classified between simple and complex. These are broken down into refined and unrefined foods.

Simple carbohydrates consist of fruits and sugars.
Refined: White sugar, fruit juice, corn syrup
Unrefined: Raw honey, pure maple syrup, fruit and freshly squeezed juice.

Complex carbohydrates consist of vegetables, legumes, and whole grains.
Refined: Bread, white rice, pasta, chips, processed foods
Unrefined: Vegetables, legumes, whole grains, brown rice

The outline above shows that the unrefined choices are the Real Food options, which will always be optimal. These carbohydrates not only contain fiber, but are filled with vitamins and minerals that our bodies cannot not make. Vitamins and minerals are essential to our well-being; they are a support for our vitality.

What about grains? We speak more about healthy grain options in our lunch chapter (page 68). Quality grains have beneficial nutrients in them. Some people feel better with lower or no grains, but others seem to do just fine including a little more. Go to our Wellness Quiz on page 50 and evaluate how you feel after eating grains.

Let's not forget the value of vegetables and remind ourselves that these are quality, anti-inflammatory, nutrient-dense carbohydrates that we want to include daily. How many servings do you currently have each day? If you have fewer than five servings of vegetables, where can you start to include another serving?

Remember that refined carbohydrates are not real foods. They are processed, depleting and add a lot of stress to our systems. Looking to create a balance in our macronutrients will be a step towards getting the nutrients our bodies need.

Q: *How can I optimize digestion?*

A few questions to ask yourself…

Do I feel heartburn?

Do I have frequent stomachaches?

Do I have bloating?

Am I regular?

Do I have a lot of stress?

A: Our diet and lifestyle habits have a large impact on digestion. Certain steps can be taken for comfort and healing.

Digestion works best in a relaxed state.

Take a deep breath and show gratitude before a meal.

Sit down while eating.

Do not rush and chew food thoroughly.

Give it a break – do not graze throughout the day.

Eat Nutritious Foods

Eat healthy greens and fiber-rich foods.

Remove refined carbohydrates and sugars (processed foods), which impair digestion.

Drink Water

Water helps remove waste and flush toxins.

Water is vital for cell integrity and nutrient absorption.

Sleep

Digestion works during this time.

Eat your last meal at least two hours before bed.

Stress Management

Stress causes inflammation and unrest. This will eventually cause digestive discomfort.

Unplug more often – do not check email or social media right before bed.

Meditation and breathing exercises are excellent stress management tools.

DIGESTION
Common Symptoms and Solutions

CONSTIPATION
(We should have a DAILY bowel movement)

WATER
Needed for transit and removal of waste and toxins.

PROBIOTICS
Adds beneficial bacteria to help regulate bowels.

FIBER
Fruits, vegetables and flax are highly beneficial.

REMOVAL OF SUGAR / PROCESSED FOODS
These foods break down, rather than build up. They cause digestion to work much harder and our system stalls.

MOVEMENT AND BREATHING
Exercise is a known aid to get our systems moving. Yoga poses, such as twists, are especially beneficial. In addition, sitting and breathing in and out can help lower stress and, in turn, allow our systems to release.

DIARRHEA
(If chronic, could also be a sign of food sensitivity or nutrient deficiency.)

PROBIOTICS
Adds beneficial bacteria to help regulate bowels.

FIBER
Psyllium, flax and hemp are fiber-rich foods and can help solidify.

REMOVAL OF SUGAR / PROCESSED FOODS
If we eat unhealthy sugars and oils, the body quickly reacts to release them from our systems. Choose Real Foods instead.

MOVEMENT AND BREATHING
Sitting and breathing in and out can help lower stress and, in turn, allow our systems to calm.

HEARTBURN

WATER
Drink one half your body weight in ounces daily. Water has many roles in our bodies and supporting digestion is one of them.

REMOVAL OF SUGAR / PROCESSED FOODS
If we eat unhealthy sugars and oils, the body quickly reacts to release them from our systems. Choose Real Foods instead.

DIGESTIVE ENZYMES OR RAW APPLE CIDER VINEGAR
Digestive supplementation to aid in better digestion during mealtime.

HOMEMADE BONE BROTH/FERMENTED FOODS
Stimulates stomach acid production (needed for breakdown of food).

GINGER
Has shown temporary relief.

BLOATING
Is another common symptom our clients have discussed with us. Our GET REAL solution is to take out sugar and processed foods, add water and enjoy our GET REAL meal plans. You will feel lighter and more energized from this transition.

Q: *What is my target heart rate?*

This is a simple formula recommend by the ACSM (American College of Sports Medicine) to let you know what your heart rate should be during exercise.[17]

(220 - AGE) .60 = lower range for target heart rate

(220 - AGE) .80 = upper range for target heart rate

Q: *What are seasonal foods, and what's in season right now?*

Eating seasonally keeps us attuned to the earth, its elements and the cycles of nature. We are blessed to live in a time where most produce can be easily achieved, regardless of the season. While this is a great convenience, it's not necessarily the best for us. Stop and think for a minute about how much better a garden fresh summer tomato tastes than one that we may get in the winter months. This is for a reason.

Eating seasonally is important first for providing the right type of fuel to protect us from the climate as our environment provides the best foods to support our health and keep us in balance. Eating seasonally is also very economical and gives us the cleanest foods possible as fewer chemicals are needed to store or ship them.

---

17 As always consult a physician before starting an exercise program.

SEASONAL FOODS

Get Real - Whatever season you are in during this transition, look through the list below and try to incorporate one new seasonal fruit and one new vegetable per week. We realize these lists are long to say the least. But picking one or two items each week is doable.

WINTER FOODS

FRUITS:
Apples
  Granny Smith
  Pippin
  Red Delicious
Cranberry
Dates
Grape
Kiwi Fruit
Kumquat
Mandarin Orange
Naval Orange
Pear
Pomegranate

VEGETABLES:
Bok Choy
Broccoli
Brussels Sprouts
Cabbage
Cauliflower
Chard
Garlic
Ginger
Jerusalem Artichoke
Jicama
Kale
Onion
Parsnip
Potato
Pumpkin
Spinach
Sprouts
Squash
  Acorn
  Butternut
  Delicata
  Spaghetti
Sweet Potato
Turnip
Yam

AUTUMN FOODS

FRUITS:
Apple
Berries
  Blackberries
  Cranberries
Date
Fig
Grape
Melon
Pear
Pomegranate
Rosehips
Tomato - Early Fall

VEGETABLES:
Bell Pepper
Broccoli
Cabbage
  Red, Green
Carrot
Cauliflower
Cucumber
Eggplant
Jicama
Leek
Lettuce
Okra
Onion
Parsnip
Potato
Pumpkin
Shallot
Spinach
Squash
  Acorn, Banana,
  Buttercup,
  Butternut, Delicata,
  Hubbard, Spaghetti
Sweet Potato
Turnip
Yam

SPRING FOODS

FRUITS:
Avocado
Date
Grapefruit
Jicama
Lemon
Lime
Loquat
Olive
Orange
Plum
Strawberry
Tangelo
Tangerine

VEGETABLES:
Artichoke
Asparagus
Beet
Bok Choy
Broccoli
Brussel Sprouts
Cabbage
Cauliflower
Celery
Chard
Chickweed
Chives
Cilantro
Collard Greens
Comfrey
Green Onions
Green Peas
Kale
Lettuce
  Butter, Green Leaf,
  Iceberg, Red Leaf,
  Romaine
Mint
Mushrooms
Spinach
Sprouts
Sugar Peas

SUMMER FOODS

FRUITS:
Apricots
Avocado
Berries
  Blackberries
  Strawberries
  Boysenberries
  Raspberries
  Strawberries
Fig
Grapefruit
Lemon
Lime
Melons
Orange
Peach
Pear
Plum
Tangelo
Tangerine
Tomato

TROPICAL FRUITS:
Banana
Guava
Mango
Papaya
Passion Fruit
Pineapple
Sapote

VEGETABLES:

Artichoke	Lettuce
Beet	Okra
Bell Pepper	Parsley
Cabbage	Radish
Celery	Rhubarb
Chile Pepper	Spinach
Chive	Squash
Cucumber	Sugar Peas
Eggplant	Watercress
Green Beans	
Green Peas	

GET REAL Q&A

Q: What is bone broth and why am I supposed to eat it?

Most everyone is familiar with the popular books Chicken Soup for Your Soul. The phrase is catchy, and it epitomizes the satisfied feeling we get after we eat a cup of our mom's chicken soup. Bone broth takes chicken soup a step further. It's a chicken soup that is made by boiling down the bones to get the most nutrients possible into a delicious broth. Bone broth may be a trend, with "shots" being sold in upscale health food stores and food trucks, but it's also a nourishing tradition with ancient roots.

We at Get Real are big fans of bone broth and this is why:
- Properly prepared bone broth is loaded with vitamins and minerals.
- Properly prepared bone broth is a great digestive aid alone or mixed in soups.
- Properly prepared bone broth is an affordable way to get quality nutrients to picky eaters. (Who doesn't like chicken noodle soup?)

Below is our personal bone broth recipe. It's a staple in both of our houses, so much so that our children request it. Give it a try or if you're not ready to start brewing your own, look for a fresh option in your local grocery store. Buying it in the store will be a bit pricier than making your own.

BONE BROTH

INGREDIENTS: organic chicken, carrots, celery, water, himalayan salt

1 whole	organic chicken remove giblets (usually a bag in cavity)	Place all ingredients in a stock pan and bring to boil, once boiling reduce to medium heat for one hour. After one hour remove chicken from stockpot and de-bone. Save chicken for later use. Place bones back into pot and continue to simmer on low heat for eight hours or overnight in crock-pot. Strain broth through a fine mesh strainer, throwing away vegetables and bones. Store broth in glass jars in refrigerator up to two weeks or the freezer for six weeks.
3 whole chopped	carrots	
2 stalks	celery	
4 quarts	pure clean water	
3 tbs	Himalayan salt	

CHICKEN NOODLE SOUP

INGREDIENTS: chicken, carrots, celery, bay leaf, bone broth, himalayan salt, butter or olive oil, noodles

3 cups cooked	shredded chicken	This really is chicken soup for your soul. Chop carrots and celery and sauté on low with butter or olive oil in a stockpot over low heat. Once soft, add broth, shredded chicken, and bay leaf and bring to a boil. Let cook for 15 minutes then add noodles and cook to package instructions. Salt and pepper to taste. Serve with a salad for a nourishing, complete meal.
10	carrots	
10 stalks chopped	celery	
1	bay leaf	
64 ounces	organic chicken broth	
4 tablespoons	Himalayan salt	
4 tablespoons	butter or olive oil	
1 package 16 oz	egg noodles	

TRANSITION MEAL PLAN #1

DAY	BREAKFAST	LUNCH	DINNER	SNACKS
MONDAY	Eggs Your Way Applegate Turkey Sausage RECIPE ON PAGE 106	Turkey and Swiss Sandwich with Crackers and Nut Butter and Apple Slices	Vegetable Soup and Grilled Cheese Sandwich RECIPE ON PAGE 134	Chocolate Cookies RECIPE ON PAGE 135
TUESDAY	Baked Pears with Cinnamon RECIPE ON PAGE 105	Leftover Soup with Crackers and Apple-sauce	Taco Night RECIPE ON PAGE 133	Peanut Butter and Oats Power Ball RECIPE ON PAGE 137
WEDNESDAY	What Happened to Our Pop Tart? Toast RECIPE ON PAGE 110	Make-Your-Own Lunch-able RECIPE ON PAGE 115	OK Enchilada Casse-role RECIPE ON PAGE 129	Smoothie RECIPE ON PAGE 109
THURSDAY	Bulgarian Yogurt and Muesli RECIPE ON PAGE 105	Wrap-It-Up Lettuce Wrap with Turkey and Avocado RECIPE ON PAGE 116	Pizza Night RECIPE ON PAGE 124	Homemade Popcorn RECIPE ON PAGE 136
FRIDAY	Smoothie (Add a Dash of Cinnamon) RECIPE ON PAGE 109	Reuben Sandwich RECIPE ON PAGE 117	Spaghetti and Greens RECIPE ON PAGE 131	Apple Sami RECIPE ON PAGE 135
SATURDAY	Apple Muffins RECIPE ON PAGE 103	BLT Salad RECIPE ON PAGE 118	Jalapeño Burgers RECIPE ON PAGE 126	Chocolate Mousse RECIPE ON PAGE 135
SUNDAY	Grab-and-Go Eggs and Bacon	Nut Butter and Honey Sandwich with Chips and Dried Apples	Orange Chicken and Rice RECIPE ONPAGE 123	Organic Cheese and Fruit

TRANSITION MEAL PLAN #2 WITH KID-FRIENDLY LUNCHES

DAY	BREAKFAST	LUNCH	DINNER	SNACKS
MONDAY	Smoothie Bowl RECIPE ON PAGE 109	Peanut Butter and Honey Sandwiches with Sliced Kiwi and String Cheese	Grilled Greek Chicken and Rice RECIPE ON PAGE 125	Popcorn with Added Cinnamon and a Few Chocolate Chips RECIPE ON PAGE 136
TUESDAY	Perfectly Baked Bacon on Sourdough With Mustard and Raw Cheddar RECIPE ON PAGE 108	Grilled Chicken Slices with Sliced Boiled Eggs, Grapes and Dipping Sauce	Chicken Pile On (Crock Pot) RECIPE ON PAGE 123	Jerky and an Apple
WEDNESDAY	Quinoa Breakfast Bake RECIPE ON PAGE 108	Bagel Bites Lunch-able with Fresh Fruit RECIPE ON PAGE 115	Swiss Steak with a Green Salad RECIPE ON PAGE 133	Trail Mix RECIPE ON PAGE 137
THURSDAY	Fruit Mix with Grain-Free Granola	Lunch-able: Club Kabobs RECIPE ON PAGE 115	Beef and Broccoli RECIPE ON PAGE 121	Berries and Honey
FRIDAY	Overnight Oatmeal RECIPE ON PAGE 108	Big Ole Potato RECIPE ON PAGE 112	Beef and Vegetable Soup RECIPE ON PAGE 122	Cookies RECIPE ON PAGE 136
SATURDAY	Make-Ahead Breakfast Burritos RECIPE ON PAGE 105	Chicken Noodle Soup with Grilled Cheese Sandwiches RECIPE ON PAGE 122	Crock Pot Ribs with Roasted Potatoes and a Green of Your Choice RECIPE ON PAGE 123	Potato Skins RECIPE ON PAGE 137
SUNDAY	Sourdough Toast with Apple Preserves and a Boiled Egg	Apple Peanut Butter Wraps with Carrots and Celery, Nuts and Two Cookies	Chicken Noodle Soup with Salad or Grilled Cheese RECIPE ON PAGE 122	Smoothie RECIPE ON PAGE 109

CLEAN MEAL PLAN #1

DAY	BREAKFAST	LUNCH	DINNER	SNACKS
MONDAY	2 Eggs with Sautéed Kale and Onion RECIPE ON PAGE 106	A Hearty Blend RECIPE ON PAGE 118	Vegetable Soup Topped with Pesto RECIPE ON PAGE 134	Apple Chips and Pumpkin Seeds
TUESDAY	Cashew Smoothie Bowl RECIPE ON PAGE 109	Leftover Vegetable Soup Topped with Pesto RECIPE ON PAGE 134	Mexican Lettuce Wraps RECIPE ON PAGE 128	A Few Almonds with Seasonal Fruit
WEDNESDAY	2 Poached Eggs Over Sautéed Chopped Broccoli and Greens RECIPE ON PAGE 106	Tuna Lettuce Wraps RECIPE ON PAGE 116	Stuffed Sweet Potato RECIPE ON PAGE 132	Trail Mix RECIPE ON PAGE 137
THURSDAY	Hemp Heart Smoothie RECIPE ON PAGE 109	Bento Box: ½ Sweet Potato, Chopped Greens, Red Cabbage, Thinly Sliced Carrots and Pumpkin Seeds	Curry Chicken with Sautéed Veggies RECIPE ON PAGE 124	Thin Rice Cake with Almond Butter
FRIDAY	Steel Cut Oats with Seasonal Fruit, Grass-Fed Butter and a Few Walnuts RECIPE ON PAGE 104	Curry Chicken With Sautéed Veggies RECIPE ON PAGE 124	Butternut Squash Soup with Kale Salad RECIPE ON PAGE 122 & 127	Hard Boiled Egg and an Orange
SATURDAY	Smashed Avocado Toast and a Hardboiled Egg RECIPE ON PAGE 104	Leftover Butternut Squash Soup with Kale Salad RECIPE ON PAGE 122 & 127	Salmon with Beet, Apple Salad, and a Bowl of Greens RECIPE ON PAGE 130	Turkey Roll-Up (If Still Hungry add More Veggies)
SUNDAY	Tropical Smoothie RECIPE ON PAGE 109	Rainbow Quinoa RECIPE ON PAGE 114	Amazing Thighs over a Bed of Arugula RECIPE ON PAGE 121	Blueberries or Apples with Cinnamon

CLEAN MEAL PLAN #2

DAY	BREAKFAST	LUNCH	DINNER	SNACKS
MONDAY	Salsa Eggs with Avocado and Mango RECIPE ON PAGE 107	Grilled Chicken Salad with Avocado Dressing RECIPE ON PAGE 111	Moroccan Lentil Soup with Sweet Potato Fries RECIPE ON PAGE 128	Apple Sprinkled with Cinnamon
TUESDAY	Chocolate, Banana, Cinnamon and Cayenne Smoothie Bowl RECIPE ON PAGE 109	Shredded Cabbage Salad with Tahini Dressing Topped with Hemp Hearts and Pumpkin Seeds RECIPE ON PAGE 119	Sweet Garlic Chicken with Broccoli and Quinoa RECIPE ON PAGE 132	Green Ginger Juice RECIPE ON PAGE 109
WEDNESDAY	Chicken Apple Sausage with Sautéed Greens and ½ Sweet Potato	Apple, Cucumber, Spinach, Avocado and Ginger Smoothie RECIPE ON PAGE 109	Salmon and Fruit Salsa with Roasted Brussels Sprouts RECIPE ON PAGE 130	Hard Boiled Egg
THURSDAY	Casey's Favorite Smoothie RECIPE ON PAGE 109	Turkey Roll-Ups with Avocado, Greens and Peppers and Seasonal Fruit RECIPE ON PAGE 117	Thai Brown Rice Bowl RECIPE ON PAGE 134	Raw Zucchini "Chips" and Salsa
FRIDAY	Oatmeal Pancakes RECIPE ON PAGE 107	Chopped Salad with Tuna, Olives, Roasted Red Pepper and Sun Dried Tomato	Grilled Chicken over Marinated Portobello, Pepper and Onion RECIPE ON PAGE 125	Nut Butter with Small Apple
SATURDAY	Bananas in Coconut Milk with Cinnamon and Walnuts RECIPE ON PAGE 105	A Little Fiesta RECIPE ON PAGE 114	Jalapeño Burger with Greens, Tomato, Cucumber and Avocado RECIPE ON PAGE 126	1 Date with a Few Walnuts
SUNDAY	Vegetable Omelets with Seasonal Fruit RECIPE ON PAGE 107	Ranbow Quinoa Bowl with Chopped Kale, Avocado and Red Onion RECIPE ON PAGE 114	Grilled Cajun Chicken, Greens with Lemon, Roasted Veggies RECIPE ON PAGE 124	Walnuts and an Apple

Breakfast

In this section, you will find a full list of breakfast recipes from our menus, including the groceries you will need to purchase or use from your staples.

We've also included a quick list of breakfast foods to have on hand that don't take any preparation. It's a short list, but have hope—several of our breakfast ideas take just five minutes or less to create!

NO-PREP BREAKFAST ITEMS FOR BUSY MORNINGS

- Applegate turkey sausage links
- Applegate chicken sausage patties
- Grain-free granola
- Pre-mixed smoothie packs (just add water)
- Grab-and-Go Eggs (a.k.a. make-ahead boiled eggs)
- Sourdough English muffins

Recipes

APPLE MUFFINS

INGREDIENTS: oats, flour, baking powder, baking soda, salt, cinnamon, vanilla, dried dates, apples, milk of choice, eggs

2 ½ cups	old fashioned oats
1 cup	dried dates
1 ½ cups	diced apple (4 apples)
¾ cup	milk (coconut, almond, cows, etc.)
2	eggs
2 teaspoons	vanilla
2 teaspoons	baking powder
½ teaspoon	baking soda
½ teaspoon	salt
½ teaspoon	cinnamon

Soak dates in water for 5 minutes. Blend oats in a blender to make into a flour. Take dates out of water. Add everything to a blender except ½ cup of the apple. Blend until smooth. Add remaining apples. Line muffin tins with parchment paper liners and fill ¾ full. Bake at 350 for 30-35 minutes.

APPLESAUCE

INGREDIENTS: apples, water, cinnamon, coconut oil

12	apples
¼ cup	water
1 tablespoon	cinnamon
1 tablespoon	coconut oil

Places apple slices in large sauce pan over low heat. Add water and cinnamon. Allow to simmer, stirring often until apples are soft (about 20 minutes).

Place apples in a blender and puree. Add coconut oil and blend just about 30 seconds. Enjoy pure fresh applesauce.

SERVES 6

AVOCADO TOAST & HARD BOILED EGGS

INGREDIENTS: bread, avocado, egg, lime, sea salt

1 - 2 hard boiled	egg
1 piece	Ezekiel or sourdough
½ small	avocado
Juice of ½	lemon or lime

Boil eggs. This usually takes about 7 minutes once a hard boil is reached (night prior is best). Toast bread, add avocado and 'smash' with fork. Add juice of lemon/lime and sea salt.

BANANA BREAD

INGREDIENTS: banana, raw honey, nut butter, eggs, coconut flour, baking soda, baking powder, cinnamon, sea salt

3 medium	bananas
1 tablespoon	raw honey
1 teaspoon	vanilla extract
¼ cup	nut butter
3	eggs
3/4 cup	coconut flour
½ teaspoon	baking soda
½ teaspoon	baking powder
½ teaspoon	cinnamon
¼ teaspoon	sea salt

Preheat oven to 375. Combine banana, honey, vanilla and almond butter. Mix well. Add in egg, blend well. Add remaining ingredients and blend well. Pour into parchment lined (or well greased) bread pan. Bake for 25 - 35 minutes.

Top with some butter or nut butter.

BANANA COOKED IN COCONUT MILK, WITH WALNUTS

INGREDIENTS: banana, coconut milk, cinnamon, walnuts

½ cup (full fat)	coconut milk	Add coconut milk and cinnamon to pan. Warm on med-low. Add banana and let simmer for 3 to 5 minutes (don't want them too soft). Pour in bowl and top with walnuts.
1 medium	banana	
¼ teaspoon	cinnamon	
6 raw crushed	walnuts*	
	* Can substitute another nut or nut butter.	

BAKED APPLES OR PEARS

INGREDIENTS: apples or pears, cinnamon

2-3 peeled, cored and sliced	apples or pears	Sprinkle fruit slices with cinnamon and arrange in a shallow baking dish. Ad ¼ cup water. Bake at 350 for 20 minutes.
¼ teaspoon	cinnamon	Enjoy, and save the rest for a snack.
		VARIATION: Top with Bulgarian yogurt or coconut cream and a drizzle of honey.

BREAKFAST BURRITOS

INGREDIENTS: eggs, turkey sausage or bacon, tortilla, salsa, raw cheddar cheese, butter

½ tablespoon	butter	Heat skillet over medium heat, melt butter. Add eggs and scramble. Once cooked remove from heat stir in sausage or bacon (already cooked). Place equal portions in each tortilla and sprinkle with cheese. Roll tortilla and enjoy or refrigerate up to three days.
6 scrambled	eggs	
4	tortillas	
4 slices	turkey sausage or bacon crumbles	
¼ cup fresh grated	raw cheddar	
	salsa for dipping (optional)	

BULGARIAN YOGURT AND MUESLI

INGREDIENTS: Bulgarian yogurt, raw honey, oats, raisins, berries, almonds

½ cup	Bulgarian yogurt	In a glass dish, layer yogurt, raw honey and then muesli mix. Let sit ten minutes or even overnight.
2 teaspoons	raw honey	
½ cup	rolled oats	VARIATIONS:
2 tablespoons	raisins	• Top yogurt with grain-free granola or a blend of nuts and seeds.
8 tablespoons	dried berries (we like blueberries)	• Top yogurt with fresh fruit.
4 tablespoons	slivered almonds	

SERVES 4

EGG AND KALE SCRAMBLE
INGREDIENTS: egg, kale, raw cheddar, butter, sea salt and pepper

2 tablespoons	grass-fed butter	Heat butter in skillet over low heat. Mix eggs, spinach, cheese, salt and pepper in a small bowl. Dump into warm skillet and scramble. Serves one.
2	eggs	
½ cup	kale	
⅛ cup grated	raw cheddar	
to taste	sea salt and black pepper	

EGG MUFFINS
INGREDIENTS: eggs, bacon, spinach, coconut oil, sea salt, black pepper

1 tablespoon	coconut oil	Heat oven to 375. Grease a muffin tin with coconut oil and set aside. Mix eggs, bacon, veggies and salt and pepper in a small mixing bowl. Pour evenly into the muffin tin and cook for 25 minutes, or until a toothpick is inserted and comes out clean.
6 large	eggs	
¼ teaspoon	sea salt	
¼ teaspoon	black pepper	
6 slices cooked and chopped	bacon	This is a great Sunday Morning Recipe that can last a few days in the fridge, or up to six weeks in the freezer.
¼ cup finely chopped	spinach or broccoli	

SERVES 6

EGGS YOUR WAY
INGREDIENTS: eggs, ghee, sea salt and pepper

1 tablespoon	ghee, butter, or coconut oil	Heat skillet over medium heat using lard. Cook eggs to your desire. Enjoy with pink salt and fresh pepper.
2	eggs	
to taste	sea salt and black pepper	

POACHED EGGS OVER SAUTÉED BROCCOLI AND GREENS
INGREDIENTS: eggs, ghee, broccoli, and kale or spinach

2	eggs	**Eggs:** Fill small pot ¾ with water and bring to a boil. Once boiling, crack two eggs into the water. Turn the heat to medium, let cook for 1 ½ - 2 minutes. Take eggs out of water with slotted spoon. Place on top of greens, add sea salt and black pepper.
1 tablespoon	ghee	
½ cup chopped	broccoli	
1 cup chopped	greens	

Broccoli and Greens: In sauté pan, add ghee and melt. Once ghee in melted, add broccoli and greens, turn to medium and sauté until softened.

SALSA EGG WITH AVOCADO AND MANGO

INGREDIENTS: eggs, salsa, avocado, butter and mango

2	eggs
3 tablespoons	salsa
1 tablespoon	butter
¼	avocado
½ cup	mango

In sauté pan, heat butter. Once warm on medium heat, add 2 eggs to scramble. Cook for 1 minute and then add the salsa. Cook until eggs are done. Serve with avocado and mango.

OATMEAL PANCAKES

INGREDIENTS: egg, rolled oats, banana, cinnamon, vanilla, butter, pure maple syrup

1 tablespoon	butter
1	egg
½ large or 1 small	banana*
½ cup	oats
¼ teaspoon	cinnamon
½ teaspoon	vanilla

* Can replace banana with unsweetened applesauce.

Place all ingredients (except syrup) in blender until it forms a thick batter. Warm butter in pan, once hot add batter to form two pancakes. Flip to finish cooking and then serve with a drizzle of pure maple syrup.

TIP: Can replace banana with unsweetened applesauce.

SERVES 1 (increase per individual)

OAT BARS

INGREDIENTS: rolled oats, nut butter, egg, raw honey, coconut oil, cinnamon, dark chocolate chips, sea salt

2 cups	rolled oats
½ cup	nut butter
1	egg
¼ cup	raw honey
1 teaspoon	cinnamon
¼ teaspoon	sea salt
¼ cup	coconut oil
⅓ cup	dark chocolate chips

Blend all ingredients together, except coconut oil and chocolate. Add melted coconut oil and then chocolate chips. Place mixture in parchment lined baking dish and spread evenly. Bake at 350 for 15-17 minutes, until edges are slightly brown.

TIP: Try to double batch and freeze half.

OMELET AND VEGGIES

INGREDIENTS: eggs, vegetables, butter or ghee, seasonal fruit

1 tablespoon	butter or ghee
2	eggs
¾ cup chopped	vegetables
	seasonal fruit

Add butter to pan and melt. Add vegetables to soften. Crack two eggs into a bowl and mix together. Pour over cooked vegetables on med-high. Let the bottom of the egg firm up and then flip ½ on top (fold in half). Let cook for 1 minute and then flip and cook for an additional minute. Serve with seasonal fruit.

OVERNIGHT OATMEAL

INGREDIENTS: oats, milk, plain Bulgarian yogurt, chia seeds, honey, cinnamon, applesauce

1/4 cup	oats (old-fashioned)	Stir all ingredients together, put into mason jar. Refrigerate overnight. Enjoy.
1/3 cup	milk (we like coconut)	
1/4 cup	plain Bulgarian yogurt	
1 teaspoon	chia seeds	OPTIONAL: Mix in cinnamon-applesauce before refrigerating.
1 teaspoon	honey	
CINNAMON APPLESAUCE:		
1/2 teaspoon	cinnamon	
1/4 cup	applesauce	

PERFECTLY BAKED BACON

INGREDIENTS: bacon

1 package	bacon (read the label)	Heat oven to 400. Line a baking dish with foil, with a wire rack on top of the foil. place sliced bacon on rack and bake for 20-30 minutes.
		TIP: Your bacon's label should say "no nitrates" and "no nitrates added."

SERVING: 2 slices of bacon per person

QUINOA BREAKFAST BAKE

INGREDIENTS: quinoa, cinnamon, almond butter, eggs, unsweetened coconut milk, vanilla, coconut oil, maple syrup, sea salt

½ teaspoon	sea salt	Bring three cups of water to boil. Add ½ teaspoon of salt, and 1 ½ cup of quinoa. Simmer for about 20 minutes or until quinoa is cooked completely (you will see little halos around each piece when it's done cooking). Allow to cool.
1 ½ cup	quinoa	
2 tablespoons	coconut oil	
2	eggs	
½ cup	unsweetened coconut milk	Meanwhile, preheat oven to 350. Grease an 8x8 baking dish with coconut oil.
1 tablespoon	vanilla	Whisk together eggs, coconut milk, vanilla, cinnamon and maple syrup. Add in cooked and cooled quinoa. Stir well and pour into greased baking dish.
1 tablespoon	cinnamon	
2 tablespoons	maple syrup	
dollop	almond butter	

Bake 25 minutes until golden. Allow to cool and cut into squares, serve with a dollop of nut butter.

SMOOTHIES / SMOOTHIE BOWLS: We like to give the name grumpy smoothie to the idea of dressing up a smoothie to distract "those" who may be a little reluctant to try smoothies. This is just a simple tip of putting your smoothie in a fun cup with a lid and silly straw. Another variation is to cover the top with a " bit" of whipped cream and add a fun straw. For more smoothie options skip to the snack section of our recipes.

INGREDIENTS: hemp seeds, almond butter, honey, frozen berries, almond milk, almond butter

2	avocados
1	banana
½ cup frozen	berries
½ cup	almond milk
2 tablespoons	hemp seeds
2 tablespoons	almond butter
2 tablespoons	honey
	fresh seasonal berries (optional)

Blend all ingredients. Pour in bowl, top with fresh berries, hemp hearts, and drizzle with honey! Serves two.

VARIATIONS:

- **Chocolate Banana:** ½ avocado, 1 frozen banana, 1 tablespoon cocoa powder, ½ cup milk of choice, 1 scoop protein powder. (Optional add in: Cinnamon)

- **Blueberry Hemp Heart:** 4 tablespoons hemp hearts, 1-2 scoops protein powder, 4 cups of spinach, 2 cups blueberries, 2 cups of ice (serves 3 - 4)

- **Cashew Smoothie:** ¼ cup cashews (soaked overnight), 1 cup frozen berries, ¼ cup water

- **Green Smoothie:** ½ small avocado, ½ cucumber, 2 handfuls spinach, ½ apple, ½ cup frozen mango, 2 scoops protein powder, ½ cup filtered water. Add in some ginger or frozen banana for variation

- **Tropical Smoothie:** 1 cup frozen tropical fruit, ⅛ tsp turmeric, crushed black pepper, ⅓ cup coconut milk, 1 - 2 scoops protein powder

- **Casey's Favorite:** ½ cup blueberries, ½ frozen banana, ⅓ cup coconut milk, 1 scoop protein powder and 2 tablespoons chia seeds

FRENCH TOAST

INGREDIENTS: bread, eggs, cinnamon, vanilla, butter or ghee, maple syrup

2 slices	Ezekiel or sourdough bread	Crack egg in bowl and whip with fork. Add cinnamon and vanilla to egg. Place toast in egg and immerse both sides (don't get soggy). Heat butter in pan and then add dipped toast to pan. Let cook for 2 minutes and then flip. Cook until firm on outside, but soft inside. Add a drizzle of pure maple syrup.
1	egg	
½ teaspoon	cinnamon	
1 teaspoon	vanilla	
1 tablespoon	butter or ghee	
drizzle	pure maple syrup	

TOAST AND NUT BUTTER

INGREDIENTS: bread, nut butter, berries, raw honey

1 slice	transitional bread	Toast bread in toaster oven. Spread nut butter over toast top with berries and drizzle honey.
1 tablespoon	nut butter per slice of toast	**TIP:** Makes a great snack too
¼ cup	berries per slice	
1 teaspoon	honey per slice	

WHAT HAPPENED TO OUR POP TART? TOAST

INGREDIENTS: bread, butter, sugar, cinnamon, seasonal fruit

¼ cup melted	real butter	Turn on oven broiler to low. Melt butter and spread on toast. Sprinkle with cinnamon and sugar. Place under broiler and watch closely.
8 slices	transitional bread	
1 teaspoon	sugar per slice	Serve with fresh fruit.
2 tablespoons	cinnamon	

SERVES 4

Lunch

The goal for lunch is always a quick fix. We have included a few weekend lunch ideas that take a little more attention, but for the most part we hope that you can make and pack these in a jiff. When making your menus for the week please check out these recipes and decide how many portions you will be making for each.

Recipes

AVOCADO DRESSING WITH CHICKEN AND SIMPLE SALAD

INGREDIENTS: avocado, lemon, cilantro, garlic, sea salt, chicken, greens, sea salt, black pepper

½ small	avocado	In blender add avocado, garlic, lemon, water and cilantro and blend well. Add sea salt and black pepper to taste.
1 small chopped	clove of garlic	
2 tablespoons	lemon	Serve over bed of greens, chopped cucumber, tomato and sliced chicken.
1-2 tablespoons	water	
2 tablespoons chopped	fresh cilantro	
1 cooked	chicken breast	
¼ chopped	cucumber	
3 halved	grape tomatoes	
1 ½ cups	greens (spinach, kale, romaine or a blend)	
to taste	sea salt & black pepper	

BACK TO BASICS: HARD BOILED EGG, RAW VEGGIES WITH GUACAMOLE, SEASONAL FRUIT

INGREDIENTS: egg, avocado or guacamole, carrots, peppers, cucumber, seasonal fruit

2 hard boiled	eggs	Pack in Bento box. Enjoy.
½ small	avocado or guacamole	
raw medley	carrots, peppers, and cucumber	
	seasonal fruit	

BIG OLE POTATOES

INGREDIENTS: russet baking potatoes, butter, bacon, raw cheddar, frozen broccoli florets, sea salt, black pepper

4 whole	russet baking potatoes	Bake potatoes. Mix cheese, cooked broccoli, bacon and butter together and disperse evenly among potatoes. Sea salt and black pepper to taste.
4 tablespoons	butter	
8 slices	perfectly baked bacon (recipe on page 108)	
1 cup	raw cheddar	
2 cups	frozen broccoli florets	SERVES 4
to taste	sea salt and black pepper	

CAPRESE WRAP

INGREDIENTS: flatbread, arugula, mozzarella, basil, tomato and kalamata olives with sea salt, black pepper

1 piece	flatbread	Place all ingredients inside flatbread and roll. Cut in half.
1 cup	arugula	
2 slices	fresh mozzarella	
3 - 4	fresh basil leaves	
3 thin slices	tomato	
5	kalamata olives	
to taste	sea salt and black pepper	

CHICKEN SALAD WITH AVOCADO AND ROMAINE ON EZEKIEL WITH SEASONAL FRUIT

INGREDIENTS: Ezekiel bread, sea salt, cooked chicken, avocado, cilantro, lime, red onion, romaine, seasonal fruit

3-4 oz cooked	chicken	Shred or dice chicken and blend with avocado, cilantro, red onion and sea salt. Place on bread, add romaine leaves and top with another piece of bread.
½ small	avocado	
juice of ½	lime	
1 tablespoons chopped	cilantro	**OPTIONAL:** Add a little cilantro and squeeze of lime juice to the chicken salad.
2 tablespoons chopped	red onion	
2 leaves	romaine lettuce	
2 slices	Ezekiel bread	
to taste	sea salt	
	seasonal fruit	

FIESTA WRAP WITH SEASONAL FRUIT

INGREDIENTS: Black Beans, flatbread wrap, avocado, tomatoes, romaine, seasonal fruit

⅓ cup	black beans	Lay out flatbread and add romaine leaves to bottom. Add avocado and 'smash' it into the lettuce. Add beans and tomatoes. Roll the wrap and cut in half.
1	flatbread	
½ small	avocado	
5	grape tomatoes	Enjoy with a side of seasonal fruit.
2 leaves	romaine lettuce	

OPTIONAL:

2 tablespoons	cilantro
2 tablespoons chopped	onion
	seasonal fruit

FUN BOWLS

INGREDIENTS: quinoa, parsley, broccoli, avocado, pumpkin seeds, extra virgin olive oil, sea salt, black pepper

½ cup	quinoa	Prepare quinoa according to package. Once done, add to bowl and top with remaining ingredients. Drizzle with extra virgin olive oil and add some sea salt and black pepper.
¼ cup chopped	parsley	
½ cup chopped	broccoli	
½ small	avocado	
3 tablespoons	pumpkin seeds	
1 tablespoon	extra virgin oilive oil	**SERVES 1** (increase per individual)
to taste	sea salt and black pepper	

QUINOA SALAD WITH SUNFLOWER SEEDS AND HEMP HEARTS, SEASONAL FRUIT

INGREDIENTS: quinoa, sunflower seeds, hemp hearts, extra virgin olive oil, cucumber, grape tomatoes, parsley, lemon, kale, sea salt

½ cup	cooked quinoa	Place cooked quinoa in bowl, add vegetables and parsley. Squeeze juice of ½ lemon over top along with extra virgin olive oil and sea salt. Add seeds blend over the top.
¼ cup	sunflower seed/hemp heart blend	
1 tablespoon	extra virgin olive oil	**OPTIONAL:** Can substitute seeds with other protein.
⅓ cup	chopped cucumber	
5 halved	grape tomatoes	
2 sprigs chopped	parsley	
juice of ½	lemon	
1 leaf finely chopped	kale	
to taste	sea salt	

RAINBOW QUINOA OR BROWN RICE

INGREDIENTS: quinoa or brown rice, red cabbage, carrots, avocado, greens, cherry tomatoes, pepitas, sunflower seeds or walnuts

½ cup	quinoa or brown rice
½ cup shredded	red cabbage
⅓ cup shredded	carrots
½ small	avocado
1 ½ cups	greens
4 halved	cherry tomatoes
optional add on:	pepitas, sunflower seeds or walnuts

Prepare quinoa. Once done add to bowl, top with all the ingredients listed to the left. Drizzle with extra virgin olive oil and add some sea salt and black pepper.

SERVES 1 (increase per individual)

A LITTLE FIESTA

INGREDIENTS: brown rice, black beans, sweet potato, romaine lettuce, grape tomatoes (or salsa), avocado

½ cup cooked	brown rice
¼ cup cooked	black beans
¼ baked	sweet potato
1 cup	chopped romaine
5 halved	grape tomatoes (can be salsa or pico)
½ small	avocado (avocado dressing works well here too)

Place cooked brown rice in bowl add the toppings and enjoy.

LUNCH-ABLE IDEAS: BASICALLY A LUNCHABLE BUT CLEAN

INGREDIENTS: crackers, white cheese, turkey slices, cucumber

6	crackers (look for 5 ingredients or less)	Simply pack it up. We like the bento box or planet box. You can find these often at discount stores.
1 oz sliced	white cheese (slice your own to save money)	
3 oz slices	turkey slices (nitrate free)	
½ cup sliced	cucumber (slices are easy for kids to incorporate)	

LUNCH-ABLE: CLUB KABOBS

INGREDIENTS: turkey, pepperoni, mozzarella cheese, bacon, tomatoes, plastic kabob sticks, honey mustard

2 oz	turkey	Cut all ingredients into bite sized pieces, except grapes and tomatoes. Slide onto kabobs. Serve with honey mustard or ranch for dipping.
5 pieces	pepperoni	
1 oz cubes	mozzarella cheese	
1 piece	bacon	
½ cup	grapes or santa tomatoes	
	plastic kabob sticks	
optional:	honey mustard	

LUNCH-ABLE: BAGEL BITES

INGREDIENTS: bagel buns, tomato sauce, fresh mozzarella, nitrate free pepperoni

4 thin	bagel buns (8 flat pieces)	Open bagels and spread a small amount of tomato sauce on each one. Sprinkle generously with cheese and pepperoni if desired. Place on cookie sheet and heat under broiler.
1 cup	tomato sauce	
2 thin slices	fresh mozzarella	For a more adventurous version add fresh spinach and mushrooms.
optional:	nitrate free pepperoni	

LUNCH-ABLE: JERKY AND CHEESE

INGREDIENTS: turkey jerky, cheese squares, grapes, carrots, celery, peanut butter, chocolate morsels

3 oz	turkey jerky	Kids love to build their own lunches. Pack all these ingredients and let them "play."
3	cheese squares	
½ cup	grapes	
¼ cup	carrots	
2 sticks	celery	
1 tablespoon	peanut butter	
1 tablespoon	chocolate morsels	

Sandwiches

HUMMUS SANDWICH

INGREDIENTS: bread, kalamata olives, lettuce, cucumber, tomato, hummus, pickles, seasonal fruit

2 slices	Ezekiel or sourdough bread	Stack all ingredients inside bread. Make sure your pickles come from the refrigerated section of the grocery store. Read the label.
2 large leaves	lettuce or arugula	
½ thinly sliced	cucumber	Enjoy with seasonal fruit.
½ thinly sliced	tomato	
5	kalamata olives	
3 tablespoons	hummus	
	seasonal fruit	

LETTUCE WRAP WITH TURKEY AND AVOCADO, SEASONAL FRUIT

INGREDIENTS: turkey, lettuce/greens, avocado, cucumber or bell peppers, seasonal fruit

4 oz cooked	turkey breast	Lay 3 - 4 pieces of turkey flat. Add avocado and lettuce to each and roll.
4 large leaves	lettuce	
½ small	avocado	Slice cucumber or bell pepper for a side along with a piece of seasonal fruit.
½	cucumber or bell pepper	
	seasonal fruit	

LETTUCE WRAP WITH TUNA

INGREDIENTS: wild tuna, red wine vinegar, sun-dried tomato, kalamata olives, roasted red pepper, Lettuce

1 can, 5 oz	wild tuna	Blend all the ingredients listed, except lettuce leaves. Add sea salt & black pepper. Place mixture in 2 large lettuce leaves.
3	sun dried tomatoes	
3 chopped	kalamata olives	Slice cucumber or bell pepper for a side.
⅛ cup	roasted red peppers	
2 tablespoons	red wine vinegar	
2-3 large leaves	lettuce or greens	

TURKEY ROLL-UPS (GREAT FOR THE LUNCH BOX)

INGREDIENTS: turkey lunch meat, mustard, provolone cheese, avocado (optional), toothpicks

3 oz	turkey lunch meat	Place a slice of turkey flat on cutting board, layer a slice of cheese on top of turkey, then a few slices of avocado or cucumber. Roll up turkey and secure with a toothpick.
1 tablespoon	mustard	
1 slice	provolone cheese	
½ small	avocado (optional)	
	toothpicks	

MEATBALL SUBS

INGREDIENTS: meatballs, lavash bread, butter, fresh mozzarella, tomato sauce

3	meatballs (recipe below)	Slice bread of choice or lie flat bread open and brush with melted butter. Heat tomato sauce in sauce pan add meatballs and allow to simmer on low until warmed. Once warm place bread on baking sheet and top with meatballs and sauce. Sprinkle with cheese and heat under broiler until cheese is melted. Top with fresh basil and serve.
1 wrap	transitional bread of choice (we like lavash)	
2 tablespoons melted	butter	
2 slices	fresh mozzarella	
¼ cup	tomato sauce	

TIP: If packing for lunch heat, wrap in quick wrap and heat at work or school.

MEATBALLS

INGREDIENTS: grass-fed beef, turkey, egg, rolled oats, garlic, flat leaf parsley, parmesan cheese, coconut oil

½ pound ground	grass-fed beef	Preheat oven to 425. Mix all ingredients together in large mixing bowl. Gently mix being careful not to over mix, this can make them tough. Drizzle oil over a large rimmed cookie sheet. Using an ice cream scoop make meatballs and place them 2 inches apart on cookie sheet. Place in oven cook for 15 minute and turn, repeating every 15 minutes for 45 minutes or until cooked all the way through.
½ pound ground	turkey (you can use all turkey)	
1 slightly beaten	egg	
½ cup	rolled oats (optional)	
2 cloves minced	garlic	
1 tablespoon	flat leaf parsley	
1/4 cup grated	parmesan cheese	
2 tablespoons	coconut oil	

Serve with pasta or on crusty bread for a sandwich.

REUBEN SANDWICH

INGREDIENTS: rye bread, butter, nitrate free roast beef, raw kraut, swiss cheese

8 slices	rye bread	Preheat oven to 350. Place rye bread on a cookie sheet and butter one side of each slice of bread. Toast for a few minutes. Once butter is melted and bread is a bit stiff pile ¼ pound of roast beef on 4 slices of bread, place ¼ cup of raw kraut on top, and top with swiss cheese. Place the other slice of rye on top and place in oven. Heat for about ten minutes or until warmed all the way through.
2 tablespoons	butter	
1 pound	nitrate free roast beef	
1 cup	raw kraut	
4 slices	swiss cheese	

TIP: Raw kraut is a natural probiotic.

Salads

A HEARTY BLEND

INGREDIENTS: red cabbage, portobello mushroom, sweet potato, sugar snap peas, salmon, extra virgin olive oil, rice wine vinegar, coconut aminos, sea salt, black pepper

⅓ cup chopped	red cabbage	Place each ingredient in different section of large bowl.
½ cooked	portobello mushroom	
½ baked	sweet potato	**DRESSING:** 1 teaspoon extra virgin olive oil, ½ tablespoon rice wine vinegar, ½ tablespoon coconut aminos, sea salt and black pepper
⅓ cup	sugar snap peas	
3 oz	protein of choice (salmon would be good here)	
DRESSING:		
1 tablespoon	extra virgin olive oil	
½ tablespoon	rice wine vinegar	
½ tablespoon	coconut aminos	
to taste	sea salt and black pepper	

BLT SALAD

INGREDIENTS: romaine hearts, eggs, bacon, raw cheddar, cucumber, shredded carrots, baby tomatoes, dressing of choice

4	romaine hearts	Create beds of lettuce. Top with remaining ingredients. Enjoy with or without dressing.
4 boiled diced	eggs	
1 pound crumbled	perfectly baked bacon (recipe on page 108)	
½ cup	raw cheddar	
1 sliced	cucumber	
¼ cup	shredded carrots	
6	baby tomatoes	
2 tablespoons	dressing of choice	**SERVES 4**

CHOPPED KALE WITH APPLES AND WALNUTS, ½ SWEET POTATO

INGREDIENTS: chopped kale, apple, walnuts, sweet potato, extra virgin olive oil, raw apple cider vinegar, dijon mustard

2 cups chopped	kale	Remove kale leaves from inner stalk. Chop and place in bowl. Add diced apple and walnuts. For dressing combine extra virgin olive oil, raw apple cider vinegar and Dijon mustard and blend well. Enjoy ½ sweet potato on side.
½ diced	apple	
8 chopped	walnuts	
½ baked	sweet potato	
1 tablespoon	extra virgin olive oil	**OPTIONAL:** Red onion, beets, cucumber, carrots
1 tablespoon	raw apple cider vinegar	
1 tablespoon	dijon mustard	

MEDITERRANEAN SALAD

INGREDIENTS: chicken, grape tomatoes, red pepper, cucumber, kalamata olives, greens, extra virgin olive oil, lemon juice, garlic powder, dried oregano, sea salt, black pepper

3 oz cooked	chicken	Place each item into different section of large bowl. Drizzle with dressing.
5 halved	grape tomatoes	
⅓ cut into strips	red pepper	
½ diced	cucumber	
4	kalamata olives	**DRESSING:** Combine extra virgin olive oil, lemon juice, garlic powder, dried oregano, sea salt and black pepper.
1 ½ cup	greens	

DRESSING:

1 tablespoon	extra virgin olive oil
juice of ½	lemon
¼ teaspoon	garlic powder
½ teaspoon	dried oregano
to taste	sea salt and black pepper

SHREDDED SLAW WITH CHICKEN AND SEASONAL FRUIT

INGREDIENTS: rice wine vinegar, sea salt, cooked chicken, red and green cabbage, carrots, green onion, tahini, lemon juice, rice wine vinegar, red chili pepper flakes, seasonal fruit

1 1/2 cups shredded	red and green cabbage	Place all of the ingredients to the left in a bowl.
½ cup shredded	carrots	**DRESSING:** Combine dressing ingredients and wisk together until well blended. Add to slaw mixture. Sea salt to taste.
2 stalks chopped	green onion	
¼ cup	pepitas and sunflower seed blend or chicken	

DRESSING:

1 tablespoon	tahini
1 ½ tablespoon	lemon juice
1 ½ tablespoon	rice wine vinegar
½ teaspoon	red chili pepper flakes
	seasonal fruit

SKIP THE RANCH ROASTED RED PEPPER DRESSING OVER MEDITERRANEAN SALAD

INGREDIENTS: roasted red peppers, garlic, balsamic vinegar, extra virgin olive oil, sea salt, kalamata olives, artichoke hearts, romaine, cucumber, tomato, red onion (optional), seasonal fruit

3 oz	protein of choice
3 pitted	kalamata olives
3 quartered	artichoke hearts
2 cups chopped	romaine lettuce
½ cup	cucumber
¼ cup	tomato
6 oz roasted	red onion (optional)

DRESSING:

1 small jar	roasted red peppers
1 clove	garlic
1 tablespoon	balsamic vinegar
1 tablespoon	extra virgin olive oil
to taste	sea salt
	seasonal fruit

Make salad with chopped romaine, cucumber tomato and onion. Add olives and few artichoke hearts.

Add protein of choice: chicken or nuts/seeds.

DRESSING: Add ingredients listed to blender and puree.

TIP: If packing lunch, bring dressing on side and add prior to eating.

SRIRACHA CHICKEN SALAD OVER GREENS

INGREDIENTS: sriracha, extra virgin olive oil, chicken, salad greens, cucumber, tomato, green onion, seasonal fruit

4 oz cooked	chicken
½ tablespoon	extra virgin olive oil
1-1 ½ tablespoons	Sriracha
2 cups	greens or romaine
½ cup	chopped cucumber
¼ cup	grape tomatoes
2 stalks chopped	green onions
	seasonal fruit

Chop chicken and blend with extra virgin olive oil and Sriracha. Make bed of greens and add cucumber and tomato. Add mixture of chicken and top with green onions. Sea salt and black pepper to taste.

TIP: Can also be served on sourdough topped with greens and raw veggies on the side.

SERVES 1

Dinner

We understand that weeknights can be tough. We have included several crock pot or make ahead recipes with this in mind. Start with just one or two this week or try some of the quick fix options from week eight. We think you will find eating from home at night to be easier than you expected.

Recipes

AMAZING THIGHS WITH PESTO AND ARUGULA

Not ready to make you own pesto yet? Check out fresh pesto options in the deli section of the grocery store.

INGREDIENTS: chicken thighs, lemon, garlic powder, Kalamata olives, arugula, fresh basil, walnuts, extra virgin olive oil, garlic, sea salt, black pepper

6-8	chicken thighs	Place thighs in baking dish and squeeze juice of the lemon over the thighs, garlic powder and S&P. Bake for 20-25 minutes at 350. Once baked place over a bed of fresh raw arugula. Top thighs with 2 tablespoons of pesto and kalamata olives.
1 cut in half	lemon	
1 teaspoon	garlic powder	
3	Kalamata olives (per person)	
½ cup	arugula (per person)	**PESTO:** Place all ingredients in blender, blend until smooth.

PESTO:

2 cups	fresh basil
¼ cup	walnuts
¼ cup	extra virgin olive oil
2 cloves	garlic
to taste	sea salt and black pepper

BEEF AND BROCCOLI

INGREDIENTS: grass-fed beef sirloin steak, broccoli, liquid aminos, dried chili pepper flakes, garlic, coconut oil, ginger

1 pound sliced thinly	grass-fed beef sirloin steak	Combine sliced beef with all ingredients* except coconut oil, let sit while you wash and prep broccoli. Once broccoli is washed and chopped, add coconut oil to a pan and heat over medium. Add beef and marinade to pan and sauté. Let simmer for 5 minutes. Add broccoli to beef mixture, cover and let simmer an additional 5 minutes. Remove lid and stir and allow to simmer on low about five more minutes. Broccoli will be a little firm.
1 ½ tablespoon	liquid aminos	
1 teaspoon dried	chili pepper flakes	
2 cloves minced	garlic	
½ tablespoon	coconut oil	
½ teaspoon fresh	ginger (optional)	
4 cups fresh	broccoli	

* Braggs liquid aminos is a soy sauce alternative, it can be found at most local grocery stores.

BEEF AND VEGETABLE SOUP crock pot friendly

INGREDIENTS: ghee, grass-fed beef stew meat, garlic, onion, tomato sauce, potatoes, carrots, green beans, beef broth, sea salt, black pepper

1 tablespoon	ghee or coconut oil
1 pound cubed	grass-fed beef stew meat
½ teaspoon minced	garlic
1 small chopped	yellow onion
1 8oz can	tomato sauce
2	potatoes
4	carrots
1 bag frozen or fresh	green beans
64 ounces	beef broth (can make or buy)
to taste	sea salt and black pepper

Heat ghee in stockpot. Add beef stew meat, garlic and onion. Sauté on low, stirring constantly until lightly brown. Meanwhile slice potatoes and carrots into bite size pieces. Stir in tomato sauce, potatoes, carrots and green beans, sea salt and black pepper. Add beef broth and let simmer one hour. Salt and pepper to taste.

TIP: To make in crock pot, just dump all ingredients and cook for 8 hours on low. This soup also freezes well.

To make beef broth follow chicken broth recipe substituting beef for chicken. Recipe found on page 98.

BUTTERNUT SQUASH SOUP

INGREDIENTS: butternut squash, onion, celery, apple, ghee, bone broth or stock, thyme, sea salt, black pepper

1 large cooked	butternut squash
1 small diced	onion
1 diced	apple
2 stalks diced	celery
1 tablespoon	ghee
2-3 cups	chicken bone broth
1 teaspoon	thyme
to taste	sea salt and black pepper

Sauté onion, apple and celery in pan with ghee. Add thyme and salt and pepper. Once mixture is softened, add broth. Simmer for 3 minutes. Add squash and mixture from pan to blender and blend well. Amount of broth depends on how thick you like it. Start with 1 cup and then slowly add more until desired thickness.

NOTE: To cook squash peel cut into 2 inch pieces. Place in steamer until tender (15-20 minutes) or roast at 375 for 30-35 minutes.

CHICKEN NOODLE SOUP

INGREDIENTS: cooked chicken, carrots, celery, bay leaf, chicken broth, sea salt, black pepper, butter, egg noodles

3 cups cooked	chicken
10	carrots
10 stalks	celery
1	bay leaf
64 ounces	organic chicken broth
4 tablespoons	sea salt
4 tablespoons	butter or olive oil
1 package 16 oz	egg noodles

This really is chicken soup for your soul. Chop carrots and celery and sauté on low with butter or olive oil in a stockpot over low heat. Once soft, add broth, chicken, and bay leaf and bring to a boil. Let cook for 15 minutes then add noodles and cook to package instructions. Salt and pepper to taste. Serve with a salad for a nourishing, complete meal.

CHICKEN PILE ON crock pot

INGREDIENTS: chicken breast, red onion, tomatoes, jalapeño, garlic, cumin, lime, chicken broth, romaine lettuce
optional: raw cheddar cheese, black beans, salsa

4	chicken breasts	Place chicken breasts in crock-pot with red onion, diced tomatoes, jalapeño, garlic, cumin, lime juice, broth and sea salt and black pepper. Allow to cook on low 6 hours. Pile chicken on bed of romaine lettuce. Optional garnishes include raw cheddar cheese, pico de gallo, black beans and salsa. Enjoy with an additional cup of warm broth.
¼ cup diced	red onion	
2 diced fresh	tomatoes (or 8oz can)	
1 whole	jalepeño	
1 clove minced	garlic	
2 tablespoons	cumin	
1 squeezed	lime	
3 cups	chicken broth	
3 hearts	romaine lettuce	

OPTIONAL: Raw cheddar cheese, black beans, salsa for toppings

CROCK POT GARLIC ORANGE CHICKEN

INGREDIENTS: Chicken thighs or drumsticks, oranges, coconut oil, liquid aminos, garlic, ginger

2 pounds	chicken thighs, breast, or drumsticks	Place chicken in crock pot, cover with remaining ingredients* and cook on low 6 hours.
1/4 cup	coconut oil	Enjoy with a side of steamed broccoli and long grain rice or rice noodles.
2 tablespoons	liquid aminos	
2 cloves minced	garlic	**TIP:** Fresh minced garlic and ginger can be found in the produce sections of most grocery stores.
3 juiced	oranges	
1 tablespoon fresh grated	ginger	

* Braggs liquid aminos is a soy sauce alternative, it can be found at most local grocery stores.

CROCK POT RIBS

INGREDIENTS: grass-fed beef ribs, minced garlic, bottled BBQ sauce, water, sea salt, black pepper

1 rack	grass-fed beef ribs (cut in half for crock pot)	Rub salt and pepper and garlic on beef. Place in crock pot with ½ BBQ sauce and water. Cook on low 6 hours. Beef will fall off bones. Serve with remaining BBQ sauce and roasted veggies.
1 clove minced	garlic	
1 bottle	quality BBQ sauce (read the label)	**TIP:** When reading label for BBQ sauce look for one with less than 4 grams of sugar per serving.
2 cups pure clean	water	
1 teaspoon	sea salt	
1 teaspoon	black pepper	

CURRY CHICKEN AND VEGETABLES

INGREDIENTS: chicken breast, cauliflower, red pepper, carrots, onion, coconut milk, bone broth or stock, coconut oil, curry powder, garlic, cayenne, sea salt, black pepper

1 tablespoon	coconut oil
1 small chopped	onion
½ head chopped	cauliflower
1 large chopped	red pepper
3 large sliced	carrots
2 tablespoons	curry powder
4 cubed bite size	chicken breasts
4 cloves minced	garlic
1 ½ cups	chicken bone broth
½ cup	coconut milk (full fat)
dash	cayenne
to taste	sea salt and black pepper

Heat pan over medium high heat and add oil. Add chicken and brown on medium high for 5 minutes (turn ½ way through). Add veggies and garlic, stir and sauté over medium heat for 5 minutes. Add curry, cayenne, salt and pepper along with the broth and coconut milk. Cover, reduce heat to low and simmer for 15-20 minutes (stir occasionally). Uncover and let sit for 5 minutes before serving.

GET REAL PIZZA

INGREDIENTS: flatbread, tomato, mozzarella, pre-made pesto, protein of choice, spinach leaves

1	flatbread of choice
½ sliced	tomato
1 ½ cups	fresh mozzarella
2 tablespoons	store bought pesto or fresh basil
4 oz	protein of choice
OPTIONAL:	
2 cups	fresh spinach leaves

Spread pesto over bread, place sliced tomato and fresh mozzarella on top of tomatoes, and sprinkle with fresh cracked pepper. Heat in broiler under low heat until cheese is melted.

PROTEIN OF CHOICE (grilled chicken, hamburger meat crumbles, prosciutto)

Enjoy with a side salad.

TIPS: Reference our bread guide on page 68 for details on choosing a flat bread. Your mozzarella should be packaged in water and choose a pesto that has a few simple ingredients.

GRILLED CAJUN CHICKEN

INGREDIENTS: chicken breast, coconut oil, cajun seasoning, coconut aminos, parsley, lemon, honey, cayenne

8	chicken breasts
⅛ cup melted	coconut oil
2 tablespoons	cajun seasoning blend
2 tablespoons	coconut aminos
¼ cup chopped	fresh parsley
1 tablespoon	raw honey
juice of 1	lemon
dash	cayenne

Place chicken in bowl. Blend all other ingredients together, mix well. Pour ingredients over the chicken and let sit for 30 minutes. Once marinated, cook on grill and serve with roasted vegetables (page 129) and greens with extra virgin olive oil and lemon juice, sea salt and black pepper.

GREEK GRILLED CHICKEN

INGREDIENTS: chicken breast, coconut oil, lemon juice, red wine vinegar, oregano, parsley, red bell pepper, zucchini, long grain rice

12	chicken breasts (if making extra for other recipes)	Long Grain Rice: Steam rice according to package, serve with butter and a bit of liquid aminos.
1 tablespoon	coconut oil	Marinate chicken breasts in melted coconut oil, lemon juice, red wine vinegar, oregano, parsley and sea salt and black pepper for at least an hour. If making kabobs quarter chicken and place on kabob sticks with red peppers, zucchini, and mushrooms.
2 tablespoons	lemon juice	
1 tablespoon	red wine vinegar	
1 ½ teaspoon	oregano	
1 teaspoon	parsley	
2 cut into big chunks	red bell pepper	Alternate cooking method: Cook full chicken breast on the grill and veggies can be roasted.
2 cut into big chunks	zucchini	Plate rice and top with grilled veggies and chicken.
16 oz fresh	mushrooms	
2 cups cooked	long grain rice	
	liquid aminos (optional)	

GRILLED CHICKEN WITH MARINATED PORTOBELLO, ONION AND PEPPER

INGREDIENTS: chicken, portobello mushrooms, red pepper, red onion, lemon, garlic, extra virgin olive oil, balsamic vinegar, crushed red pepper flakes

2 large cleaned and sliced thin	portobello mushrooms	Marinate mushrooms in olive oil, balsamic vinegar, sea salt and black pepper. Let sit for at least 30 minutes (can make in morning and marinate all day, too).
1 sliced thin	red pepper	
1 sliced thin	red onion	
3 tablespoons	extra virgin olive oil	Marinate chicken in garlic, juice of lemon, and crushed red pepper and let sit at least 15 minutes.
3 tablespoons	balsamic vinegar	

CHICKEN:

4	chicken breasts	Grill chicken. Top with portobello salad and enjoy. This also goes well over a bed of raw spinach.
2 cloves minced	garlic	
juice of 1	lemon	
½ tablespoon	crushed red pepper flakes	

HOMEMADE FRIES

INGREDIENTS: potato, coconut oil, onion powder, garlic powder, sea salt, black pepper

4	potatoes
2 tablespoons melted	coconut oil
1 teaspoon	onion powder
1 teaspoon	garlic powder
to taste	sea salt and black pepper

Cut potatoes into thick 'steak' fries. Place in bowl and pour melted coconut oil over fries. Add seasonings and mix well. Place on parchment lined baking sheet and bake at 425 for 20 minutes. Flip over and bake an additional 10 minutes.

JALAPEÑO BURGER WITH GREENS, TOMATO, CUCUMBER AND AVOCADO

INGREDIENTS: grass-fed beef, jalapeño, avocado, cucumber, romaine, cilantro, lime, garlic, sea salt, black pepper

1 pound ground	grass-fed beef or turkey
2 sliced	jalapeños,
1 large sliced	1 onion
4 - 5 cups	greens
10	grape tomatoes
1 - 2	cucumbers
2 small	avocados
½ bunch chopped	cilantro
2 tablespoons	avocado dressing

Form patties out of beef or turkey. Sauté burger in pan over medium high heat with coconut oil or ghee. Flip the burgers after 3 minutes, and add sliced jalapeño and onion. Cook an additional 5 minutes or until vegetables are tender.

In a bowl, place greens, tomato, cucumber, avocado and cilantro.

AVOCADO DRESSING: Place ingredients in blender and blend well.

SERVES 1

AVOCADO DRESSING:

½ small mashed	avocado
1 clove minced	garlic
juice of ½	lime
1 tablespoon	water
1 tablespoon chopped	fresh cilantro
to taste	sea salt and black pepper

KALE SALAD

INGREDIENTS: kale, beet, walnuts, apple, extra virgin olive oil, lemon, rosemary, sea salt, black pepper

2 cups chopped	kale
½ large cooked	beet
¼ cup	walnuts
½ thinly sliced	apple
1 tablespoon	lemon vinaigrette

LEMON VINAIGRETTE:

1 tablespoon	extra virgin olive oil
2 tablespoons	lemon juice
1 teaspoon chopped	fresh rosemary
	sea salt and black pepper

Place whole beet in 400 degree oven and bake for 1 hour until fork goes into beet. Let cool. Peel the skin and then slice. (Don't worry; the red on your hands will wash off with soap and water.)

Mix together all ingredients, and dress with lemon vinaigrette.

LEMON VINAIGRETTE: Whisk all ingredients together.

SERVES 1

LEMON CHICKEN

INGREDIENTS: chicken breast, sea salt, black pepper, butter, chicken broth, lemon, asparagus

4 boneless skinless	chicken breasts
2 tablespoons	sea salt
1 tablespoon	pepper
4 tablespoons	butter
¼ cup	chicken broth
1	lemon
2 bunches fresh washed & trimmed (frozen is an alternative)	asparagus

Heat skillet over medium heat. Season chicken with salt and pepper. Heat butter in skillet. Once melted, add seasoned chicken breast, sauté about 2 minutes on each side. Turn heat to low and add broth, cover and allow to simmer about ten minutes, turning as needed so that chicken does not stick to pan. After ten minutes, squeeze lemon juice over chicken. Toss lemon halves into pan for added flavor (remove before serving). Add fresh asparagus, allow to cook another ten minutes, covered.

MEXICAN LETTUCE WRAPS

INGREDIENTS: grass-fed beef, onion, romaine, avocado, lime, cumin, paprika, chili powder, cayenne

1 pound	grass-fed beef or ground turkey
1 small chopped	onion
1 teaspoon	cumin
1 teaspoon	paprika
1 teaspoon	chili powder
dash	cayenne
1	lime
8 big	leaves romaine
OPTIONAL:	
	guacamole
	salsa

Sauté ground meat and chopped onion. Season with cumin, paprika, chili powder and a dash of cayenne. Drain liquid. Add the lime juice.

Serve on two giant lettuce leaves and top with guacamole and salsa.

SERVES 4

MOROCCAN LENTIL SOUP

INGREDIENTS: green lentils, cauliflower, onion, carrots, bone broth or stock, coconut oil, garlic, ginger, turmeric, garam masala, cumin, cayenne, sea salt and black pepper

1 large chopped	onion
3 cloves minced	garlic
1 teaspoon grated	ginger
1 tablespoon	coconut oil
1 ½ cups	green lentils
1 can 15 oz diced	tomatoes
3 large sliced	carrots
½ head diced	cauliflower
1 teaspoon	turmeric or curry powder
1 teaspoon	garam masala
½ teaspoon	cumin
2 dashes	cayenne
4 - 5 cups	vegetable broth (depends on desired thickness)
to taste	sea salt and black pepper

In stock pot, sauté onion, garlic, ginger in coconut oil. Add broth, green lentils, diced tomatoes, sliced carrots, cauliflower, garam masala, curry or turmeric, cumin and 2 dashes of cayenne. Simmer until lentils and veggies are cooked (30 minutes). Puree half of the soup in blender. Return blended mixture to pot, stir and serve.

OK ENCHILADA CASSEROLE

INGREDIENTS: ground grass-fed beef, boxed enchilada sauce, boxed mushroom soup, corn tortillas, raw cheddar

1 pound ground	grass-fed beef or turkey	Heat oven to 350 degrees. Sauté meat until no longer pink. Add enchilada sauce and mushroom soup to the meat. Heat and stir. Meanwhile, cut all tortillas into quarters. Dip in sauce mixture and place in baking dish. Continue this until all sauce and tortillas are used. Top with fresh shredded raw cheddar and cover. Freeze at this point or cook for 20 minutes.
1 box 16 oz	enchilada sauce	
1 box 16 oz	organic mushroom soup	
15	all-corn tortillas	
shredded	raw cheddar	

POTATO SMASH

INGREDIENTS: 1

12	red bliss potatoes	Bring water to a boil and add potatoes. Let boil for 10 minutes. Remove from water and place in baking dish. Using a large spoon, place on top of potato and press down to 'smash'. Top with melted ghee, and spices. Bake in 400 degree oven for 15-20 minutes.
1 ½ tablespoon melted	ghee	
1 teaspoon	onion powder	
1 teaspoon dried	chives	
to taste	sea salt and black pepper	

ROASTED POTATOES

INGREDIENTS: red potatoes, ghee, sea salt, black pepper

¼ cup	ghee	Heat oven to 400. Melt ghee in dutch oven, toss potatoes with ghee until lightly coated. Season heavily with salt and pepper. Bake in Dutch oven for 30 minutes, stirring every ten minutes. Potato skins will get a bit crunchy.
2 pounds	red potatoes	
	sea salt and black pepper	

ROASTED VEGETABLES WITH RED BLISS POTATOES

INGREDIENTS: Red bliss potatoes, asparagus, red pepper, cauliflower, coconut oil, garlic powder, onion, sea salt, black pepper

4 quartered	red bliss potatoes	Cut asparagus into 1 ½ inch pieces. Cut red pepper into strips. Cut cauliflower into bite size pieces.
½ bunch cut	asparagus	
1 large cut	red bell pepper	Blend with melted coconut oil, garlic powder, onion powder, sea salt and black pepper. Bake at 375 degrees for 40 minutes. (Stir at 20 minutes.)
¼ head cut	cauliflower	
2 tablespoons melted	coconut oil	
1 tablespoon	garlic powder	
1 tablespoon	onion powder	
to taste	sea salt and black pepper	

SALMON WITH BEET AND APPLE SALAD, BOWL OF GREENS

INGREDIENTS: salmon, beets, apple, lemons, red onion, greens

4 fillets	Salmon
1 large thin sliced	beet
1 medium thin sliced	apple
3	lemons
½ cup thin sliced	red onion
6 cups	greens (arugula is good)

Preheat oven to 400. Place salmon fillets in roasting pan. Top salmon with thinly sliced lemons (2 per fillet), thinly sliced red onion and add sea salt. Bake for 10 - 12 minutes.

Thinly slice beets and apples and place in bowl. Add the juice of 1 lemon and sea salt.

Place greens on plate, squeeze a bit of lemon zest and juice. Top with salmon and red onions, discard the cooked lemon.

SALMON WITH FRUIT SALSA

INGREDIENTS: salmon, greens, garlic, pineapple, kiwi, mango, red onion, cilantro, cumin, jalapeño, lime, garlic, sea salt, black pepper

4 Fillets	Salmon
2 cloves minced	garlic
6 cups	green of your choice (Kale, Spinach, Arugula)
juice of 1	lime

FRUIT SALSA:

juice of 1	lime
1 ½ cups cubed	pineapple
½ cup cubed	kiwi
½ cup cubed	mango
¼ cup finely chopped	red onion
2 tablespoon	cilantro
1 teaspoon	cumin
1 chopped	jalapeño

Season salmon with minced garlic, lime juice, sea salt and black pepper. Bake salmon for 15 minutes at 400.

FRUIT SALSA: Blend together, cubed pineapple, kiwi, mango, red onion, fresh cilantro, cumin, chopped jalapeño, S&P. Squeeze juice lime over mixture and blend well.

Place salmon on bed of greens and top with hearty serving of fruit salsa.

SERVES 4

SAVORY BAKED CHICKEN LEGS

INGREDIENTS: grass-fed butter, savory spice blend, chicken legs

6	chicken legs	Heat oven to 375 degrees, place chicken in baking dish, sprinkle with spice blend, brush with butter. Cook for 45-60 minutes. Serve with a green salad and potato smash (page 129).
1-2 tablespoons	butter	
2 tablespoons	savory spice blend	

SAVORY SPICE BLEND:		
1 teaspoon	thyme	SAVORY SPICE BLEND: We like to blend thyme, onion powder, paprika, rosemary, sea salt, black pepper. Keep in a jar and it is ready to be used.
1 teaspoon	onion powder	
1 teaspoon	paprika	
1 teaspoon	rosemary	
1 teaspoon	sea salt	
½ teaspoon	black pepper	

SLOW COOKED GRASS-FED BEEF FOR FAJITAS

INGREDIENTS: garlic, chili powder, cumin, pot roast, onion, fresh jalapeño, chicken broth, fresh salsa, tortillas

1 medium	grass-fed beef pot roast	Combine all ingredients in a crock pot and cook on low for 6 hours. Grass-fed beef should shred with a fork. Quartering vegetables gives you the flavor and nutrients from cooking without actually putting an onion or jalapeño on the plate.
1 small quartered	yellow onion	
4 tablespoons fresh minced	garlic	Fill tortillas with mixture, top with cheese or salsa. Want to skip the tortilla? Enjoy over a bed of greens.
4 tablespoons	chili powder	
2 tablespoons	cumin	This is a great busy day recipe, it stays hot and can be served in rounds.
1 fresh whole	jalapeño	
32 ounces	water or chicken stock	TIPS: Fresh salsa means that it can spoil after a few days. Can be store-bought, just check for one with no sugar in the ingredients.
to taste	fresh salsa	
12	tortillas	Cumin: If you are not ready to buy all the seasonings, try buying a ready made organic taco mix.

SPAGHETTI

INGREDIENTS: garlic, extra virgin olive oil, two jars of organic pasta sauce, grass-fed ground beef or turkey, fresh basil, can of chopped black olives, spaghetti

2 jars 16 oz	organic pasta sauce	Sauté ground grass-fed beef or turkey. Add garlic, sea salt and black pepper. Cook until no longer pink. Add 2 jars of organic pasta sauce. Meanwhile, boil noodles according to instructions. Mix prepared spaghetti with a bit of olive oil. Plate noodles, top with meat sauce and olive and basil confetti.
1 pound ground	grass-fed beef or turkey	
2 tablespoon minced	garlic	
1 tablespoon	fresh chopped basil	
1 can chopped	olives	
1 package	spaghetti	
	extra virgin olive oil	

STIR FRY RICE, GINGER CHICKEN AND FROZEN VEGGIES

INGREDIENTS: chicken breast, brown rice, frozen vegetable blend (broccoli, cauliflower and carrots), ginger, coconut oil, coconut aminos, garlic, dried chili pepper flakes

4 cut into strips	chicken breasts	Place coconut oil in pan and heat. Add fresh ginger and garlic, let cook for 2 minutes on medium. Add chicken strips. Let simmer for 5-7 minutes. Add bag of frozen vegetables, coconut aminos, dried chili pepper flakes if using. Cover and let cook for 5-7 minutes. Serve over rice.
2 cups cooked	brown rice	
1 bag 16 - 20 oz	frozen veggies (broccoli, cauliflower and carrots)	
1 tablespoon	coconut oil	
1 inch fresh minced	ginger	
2 cloves minced	garlic	
3 tablespoons	coconut aminos	
1 teaspoon	red pepper flakes (optional)	

STUFFED SWEET POTATO

INGREDIENTS: sweet potato, red lentils, cauliflower, coconut oil, tomato paste, coconut milk, curry powder, garam masala, garlic powder, cayenne, sea salt and black pepper

1 medium	sweet potato	Bake sweet potato at 375 for 45 minutes in baking pan.
¼ cup dry	red lentils	Place lentils in boiling water and cook for 10 -15 minutes. In separate sauté pan add chopped cauliflower and 1 tsp coconut oil and sauté for 5 minutes. Add tomato paste, coconut milk and spices, blend well. Bring to a low boil and then let simmer until cauliflower is tender. Pour thickened sauce over sweet potato and ½ cup lentils.
1 cup chopped	cauliflower	
1 teaspoon	coconut oil	
1 tablespoon	tomato paste	
¼ cup full-fat	coconut milk	
1 teaspoon	curry	
1 teaspoon	garam masala	
1 teaspoon	garlic powder	
dash	cayenne	
to taste	sea salt and black pepper	

SERVES 1

SWEET GARLIC CHICKEN WITH BROCCOLI AND QUINOA

INGREDIENTS: chicken, garlic, ghee, honey, broccoli, quinoa

4 breasts	chicken	Preheat oven to 375. Place chicken in baking dish. In saucepan melt ghee and honey, add the minced garlic. Once melted pour over chicken and bake for approximately 15 minutes.
5 cloves minced	garlic	
2 tablespoons	ghee	
2 tablespoons	honey	Steam broccoli and flavor with coconut aminos and serve with ½ cup quinoa.
4 cups	broccoli	
2 cups cooked	quinoa	

SWISS STEAK

INGREDIENTS: extra virgin olive oil, grass-fed beef round steak, stewed tomatoes, celery, carrots, red potatoes, sea salt, black pepper

2 pounds	grass-fed beef round steak	Heat oil over medium/low heat in a large skillet or soup pan. Cut steak into quarter-sized pieces, and salt and pepper. Place in skillet allowing to sear on both sides, but not cook all the way through, about 2 minutes on each side. Remove from pan, leave drippings in pan and add in onions, carrots, and celery. Stir until onions are translucent. Add in remaining ingredients and bring to a low boil. Stir often. Once dish reaches a boil, reduce heat to low, add meat back in and cover. Allow to cook 20 minutes, stirring every 10 minutes, or until potatoes are soft. Enjoy.
1 can 16 oz	stewed tomatoes with basil, oregano and garlic	
¼ cup chopped	onion	
2 tablespoons	extra virgin olive oil	
2 stalks chopped	celery	
4 whole peeled and sliced	carrots	
4 peeled and sliced	red potatoes	
1 cup pure clean	water	
to taste	sea salt and black pepper	

TACO NIGHT

INGREDIENTS: chili powder, garlic powder, cumin, ground grass-fed beef or turkey, raw cheddar, pico de gallo, cilantro, romaine or taco shells

2 pounds ground	grass-fed beef or turkey	Sauté the meat until pink is gone. Drain any excess fluid. Add chili powder, garlic, and cumin (or taco mix if using). Fill romaine shells or taco shells with meat. Top with cheese, pico de gallo, and cilantro. Enjoy!
2 tablespoons	chili powder	
½ teaspoon	garlic powder	
½ teaspoon	cumin	
	romaine leaves or taco shells	
shredded	raw cheddar	
chopped	cilantro	
	pico de gallo	

THAI VEGGIE BROWN RICE BOWL

INGREDIENTS: brown rice, garbanzo beans, zucchini, carrot, yellow and red pepper, sugar snap peas, lime, coconut aminos, dried chili pepper flakes

2 cut into strips	zucchinis
1 large cut into strips	carrot
1 cut into strips	yellow bell pepper
1 cut into strips	red bell pepper
3 finely sliced	scallions
1 cup chopped	sugar snap peas
1 tablespoons	dried red chili pepper flakes
¾ cup full-fat	coconut milk
Juice of 2	limes
4 tablespoon	coconut aminos
2 cups cooked	garbanzo beans
.1 cup cooked	brown rice

Chop all vegetables - set aside. Prepare sauce - combine coconut milk, lime juice, coconut aminos*, chili pepper flakes and sea salt - add to pan. Allow sauce to warm on medium and add all the vegetables. Cover and simmer for approximately 7 minutes (want veggies to stay crisp).

Place ½ cup brown rice and ½ cup garbanzo beans in bowl. Top with veggies and sauce.

TIP: Make extra for lunch

SERVES 4

* Coconut aminos: This is a soy free, gluten free alternative to soy sauce. The only ingredients in the product are organic coconut tree sap and sea salt.

VEGETABLE SOUP

INGREDIENTS: carrots, onion, green or red bell pepper, green beans, broccoli, cauliflower, tomato paste, fire roasted diced tomato, bone broth or stock, bay leaf, basil, garlic, optional: chicken, quinoa, lentils or garbanzo beans or pesto

2 tablespoons	coconut oil or red palm oil
4 chopped	carrots
½ chopped	onion
3 cloves minced	garlic
1 large chopped	green or red bell pepper
1 ½ cups frozen	green beans
1 ½ cups chopped	broccoli (frozen or fresh)
1 ½ cups chopped	cauliflower (frozen or fresh)
1	bay leaf
1 ½ tablespoons	dried basil
2 tablespoons	tomato paste
1 can 15 oz	fire-roasted tomatoes
6-7 cups	chicken bone broth (can use water)

OPTIONAL:

	cooked chicken
	lentils
	garbanzo beans
	pesto

Coat stockpot with oil and warm on medium heat. Add carrots, onion and garlic and sauté for 4 minutes. Add pepper, sauté for 2 minutes. Add green beans, broccoli and cauliflower and sauté. Add red pepper flakes, bay leaves, basil and tomato paste, stir and blend. Add fire-roasted tomatoes and broth. Stir, cover and turn heat to medium low. Let simmer on your stovetop for 35 - 40 minutes. Turn off the heat and let sit for ten minutes. Season with sea salt and black pepper if you wish. Top with optional add ins or serve with cooked quinoa.

TIP: Tastes even better the next day and freezes well.

SERVES 6 GENEROUSLY

Snacks

Snacks can be tricky; it's actually the place we have to revisit the most with our families. It's easy to find yourself or your kids hungry and reaching for the quickest "fix" available. We have included some of our "go-to" snack options. We would also like to remind you if you find yourself hungry often between meals you may want to revisit our information about balanced meals on page 15 and see if you need to alter your macronutrients a bit.

Recipes

APPLE SAMI

INGREDIENTS: apples, almond butter, honey

4 large peeled and cored	apples	Peel and Core Apples. Slice in thick rounds- it should look like a bagel. Spread nut butter over apple, drizzle with honey and top with another apple.
1 tablespoon	almond butter per sami	
to taste	honey	Have fun with this you can add mini chocolate morsels or granola for a little extra crunch.

CHOCOLATE COOKIES

INGREDIENTS: organic peanut butter, honey, sugar, egg, cocoa powder, chocolate chips, sea salt

1 cup	organic peanut butter	Preheat oven to 350. Blend all ingredients well. Roll into golf ball size rounds, place on parchment lined baking sheet and and then press into cookie. Bake for 16-18 minutes. Let cool 5 minutes before serving.
¼ cup	honey	
¼ cup	sugar	
1	egg	OPTIONAL ADD IN: 1/4 cup dark chocolate chips
½ teaspoon	vanilla	
2 tablespoons	cocoa powder	
¼ cup	chocolate chips	

CHOCOLATE MOUSSE

INGREDIENTS: banana, avocado, cacao powder, coconut milk, hemp hearts

1 frozen	banana	In food processor, blend all ingredients (except hemp hearts) together. Scoop mousse into bowl and sprinkle with hemp hearts.
½ small	avocado	
1 tablespoon	cacao powder	
3 tablespoon	coconut milk	
1 tablespoon	hemp hearts	

COCONUT BITES
INGREDIENTS: egg whites, honey, sea salt, unsweetened coconut flakes

2 large	egg whites	Using a hand blender, whisk first three ingredients together until peaks form. Stir in coconut flakes and refrigerate for 30 minutes. Heat oven to 350. Line a baking sheet with parchment paper. Using an ice cream scooper create small balls, use your hands to tighten them. Place on baking sheet and cook for 10 minutes. Store in refrigerator.
¼ cup	honey	
¼ teaspoon	on sea salt	
2 ½ cups	unsweetened coconut flakes	

HOMEMADE POPCORN
INGREDIENTS: coconut oil, organic popcorn, grassfed butter, sea salt

3 tablespoons	coconut oil	In large stock pot melt coconut oil. Once melted, add the popcorn and cover. Keep on medium to medium high heat. The popcorn will start popping quickly and fill the stock pot. Once it rises to the cover, turn off heat. Melt butter. Pour popcorn in large bowl and add sea salt and butter. Blend well.
1 ½ cups	organic popcorn	
3 tablespoons	grass-fed butter	
	sea salt	

'ICE CREAM'
INGREDIENTS: frozen fruit, coconut milk

1 cup frozen	fruit	Blend well in food processor or blender until thick and creamy.
2-3 tablespoons	coconut milk	
OPTIONAL:	protein powder	

OATMEAL COOKIES no bake
INGREDIENTS: butter, raw nut butter, coconut milk, rolled oats, honey

½ cup	butter	Melt butter in a large sauce pan, add coconut milk and honey. Bring to a rolling boil. Remove from heat. Add nut butter and oats stirring quickly. Drop by spoonfuls onto wax paper and cool.
½ cup	raw nut butter	
½ cup	coconut milk	
3 cups	rolled oats	
3 tablespoons	raw honey	

PEANUT BUTTER OAT BALLS

INGREDIENTS: peanut butter, rolled oats, hemp hearts, dark chocolate chips

1 cup	peanut butter (any nut butter can be used)	Place all ingredients except chocolate in food processor. Blend well. Add chocolate and pulse a few times. Roll into 1 ½ inch balls and refrigerate.
¾ cup	rolled oats	
¼ cup	hemp hearts (can also use chia)	
¼ cup	cacao nibs or dark chocolate chips	

POTATO SKINS

INGREDIENTS: potatoes, bacon, raw cheddar, chives, coconut oil

6 sliced	potatoes	Heat oven to 350. Wash 6 medium potatoes, and slice into disks. Place in bowl and toss liberally with warm coconut oil, place potato disks on a baking sheet and bake about 15 minutes or until skins are golden, remove from oven salt and pepper to taste, sprinkle with bacon crumbles and raw cheddar. Return to oven and heat until cheese is melted. Watch closely.
1 pound	perfectly baked bacon	
1 cup	raw cheddar	
	fresh chives	
	coconut oil	
	sea salt and black pepper	

TRAIL MIX

INGREDIENTS: nuts of choice, apple chips, coconut chips, raisins, dark chocolate

1 cup	nut of choice	Mix all ingredients together and snack.
1 cup	apple chips	
½ cup	coconut chips	
½ cup	raisins or apricots	
¼ cup	dark chocolate morsels	

Dipping Sauces: Dipping sauces can be made quickly in small portions. At our houses we just add a bit of each and blend.

HONEY MUSTARD

mustard honey	Mix mustard and raw honey to desired sweetness.

FRUIT DIP

Bulgarian yogurt honey cinnamon	Mix Bulgarian yogurt, honey and cinnamon, this will be runny.

EASY RANCH

1 packet	organic ranch seasoning	Buy organic ranch seasoning packet and mix with 2 cups of Bulgarian yogurt.
2 cups	Bulgarian yogurt	

INDEX

RECITE INDEX

RECIPE INDEX

Sources

Ballantyne, Sarah. *The Paleo Approach, Reverse Autoimmune Disease and Heal Your Body*. Las Vegas: Victory Belt Publishing, 2013.

Batmanghelidj, F. *Your Body's Many Cries for Water*. USA: GHS, Inc., 1992.

Bland, Jeffrey. *Clinical Nutrition, A Functional Approach*. Washington: IFM, 2004.

Campbell-McBride, Natasha. *Put Your Heart in Your Mouth*. United Kingdom: Cambridge, England: Medinform Publishing, 2007.

Campbell-McBride, Natasha. *GAPS, Gut and Psychology Syndrome*. Cambridge, England: Medinform Publishing, 2010.

Davis, William. *Wheat Belly*. New York: Rodale Books, 2011.

Dufty, William. *Sugar Blues*. Pennsylvania: Chilton Book Co, 1975.

Enig, Mary. *Know Your Fats*. Bethesda, MD: Bethesda Press, 2000.

Fallon, Sally. *Nourishing Traditions*. Washington, DC: New Trends Publishing, 1999.

Fife, Bruce. *The Detox Book*. Colorado Springs: Piccadilly Books, 1997.

Haas, Elson. *Staying Healthy with Nutrition*. New York: Crown Publishing Group, 2006.

Jacob, Aglaee. *Digestive Health with Real Food*. Paleo Media Group, 2013

Lipski, Elizabeth. *Digestive Wellness*. McGraw Hill, 2012

Lustig, Robert H. *Fat Chance*. New York: The Penguin Group, 2012.

Malone, Linda. *ACSM Fit Society*. American College of Sports Medicine, Winter 2009.

Murray, Michael and Pizzorno, Joseph and Pizzorno, Laura. *The Enclyclopedia of Healing Foods*. New York: Atria Books, 2005.

Murray, Michael T. and Pizzorno, Joseph. *The Encyclopedia of Natural Medicine.* New York: Atria Paperback, 1998.

Rossy, Lynn. *The Mindfulness-Based Eating Solution.* Oakland, NewHarbinger Publications, Inc., 2016.

Sanfilippo, Diane. *Practical Paleo.* Victory Belt Publishing, 2012.

Tortora, Gerald and Derrickson, Bryan. *Introduction to the Human Body.* New York: John Wiley & Sons, Inc., 2010.

Wansink, Brian. *Slim by Design: Mindless Eating Solutions for Everyday Life.* Harper Collins, 2014.

Weatherby, Dicken. *Signs and Symptoms Analysis from a Functional Perspective.* Bear Mountain Publishing, 2004.

Wright V., Jonathan and Lenard, Lane. *Why Stomach Acid is Good for You.* Maryland: M. Evans, 2001.

About the Authors

MARY PRATT, BCHN, NTP, 500 HR RYT

Mary studied nutrition with the Nutritional Therapy Association and became certified in June 2014. She became board certified through the NANP as a Holistic Nutritionist in April of 2015. Mary practices with groups and individual clients through her business, beNourished. In addition to her nutrition background, Mary has been practicing and studying yoga for seven years and teaches a mindfulness-based practice in her classes. (She was trained through Freelife people.) Mary believes the key to wellness is to tune into your choices, choose real foods, notice your body's response and support this lifestyle on a daily basis.

Mary is married to Rich Pratt, a recently retired Army officer, and has spent the past 20 years supporting the military community. Together, they have three boys aged 17, 15 and 13. Her family has been extremely supportive in her career and has tested countless recipes for her to bring into practice. Mary is a native Bostonian.

For more information, visit www.benourishedwellness.com

AMY YATES, BS, NTP

Amy has always had a passion to help others understand the connection between spiritual, emotional and physical health. She has spent more than 15 years in the health and fitness industries, working in hospitals, schools and churches.

Amy did her undergraduate work at Abilene Christian University in Abilene, TX and her graduate work at Baylor University, in Waco, TX. She is certified by the Nutritional Therapy Association and the American College of Sports Medicine. Amy has numerous group fitness certifications and serves as a health adviser on both local and state boards. She has a private nutrition practice in Abilene, TX. Amy's compassion and knowledge combine in a unique way to empower her clients to truly become the healthiest "selves" they can be.

Amy currently lives in Clyde, TX with her husband, Jerod, and their three children, Allie, Landon and Kate.

For more information, visit TheGroceryGirl.com

Acknowledgments

We would like to express our gratitude to those who provided support, guidance, love, tasting, critique and patience to us as we embarked on this adventure.

We would not have had the words or motivation without the support of each other as we outlined, brainstormed, shared and laughed through the process. We started out as colleagues and ended up as friends and that itself is enough.

To our husbands, thank you for being sounding boards, giving us space and supporting us in countless ways on this journey. You have played such big roles from beginning to end, in the ways you have believed in us, empowered us and kept us motivated to complete this project.

We would both like to thank our kids who have gone through the Get Real transition and are all still nothing but supportive. They have been our taste tasters on a daily basis. We are grateful for all of your recommendations along the way; each one of you has a place in this book and your openness in the journey has been priceless.

We would like to send an extra special thanks to our editor, Nicole Bowman who has an amazing skill to blend two different authors and make our voices one. We are grateful for your skill, patience and suggestions.

Our next extra special thanks goes to our graphic designer Christine Gors who has the amazing skill to bring our words to life. We know that each reader will have a better understanding of our work due to your creative abilities. Thank you.

There are many other family members, friends and colleagues to thank. We appreciate each of you and the roles you have played.

Love,

Amy and Mary